On Sight & Insight

90 0476931 4

On Sight
& Insight

a journey into the world of blindness

John M. Hull

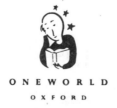

ONEWORLD
OXFORD

ON SIGHT AND INSIGHT
A JOURNEY INTO THE WORLD OF BLINDNESS

Oneworld Publications
(Sales and Editorial)
185 Banbury Road
Oxford OX2 7AR
England

Some of the material in this book was previously published as
Touching the Rock: An Experience of Blindness
by SPCK

© John M. Hull 1990, 1997
Reprinted 2001

All rights reserved
Copyright under Berne Convention
A CIP record for this title is available
from the British Library

ISBN 1–85168-141-8

Cover design by Peter Maguire
Printed and bound by WS Bookwell, Finland

UNIVERSITY OF PLYMOUTH
LIBRARY SERVICES

Item No.	9004769314
Class No.	
Contl No.	1851681418

To Marilyn
and to
Imogen, Thomas, Elizabeth,
Gabriel and
Joshua

Contents

Foreword

In 1983, three years after I became a registered blind person, I began to keep a cassette diary in which I recorded my experiences. After three or four years, I had collected a considerable amount of material. I kept the diary partly in order to monitor my own reactions to blindness, and thus to keep some sense of balance and control in what was a deeply disturbing period of my life, and partly in an attempt to communicate with sighted people. For me, going blind had been an experience of isolation and marginalization, and I wanted to explain myself to the sighted world. I wanted the changes which had come over me and my life to become intelligible to my friends by helping them to have insight into blindness.

I had the recorded diary turned into a print transcript and arranged it into chapters. The result was *Touching the Rock: An Experience of Blindness*, published in 1990. The book went through six English language editions, not only in the United Kingdom, but also in America and Australia. Michael Burke produced a forty-minute film on the book which was first broadcast on June 2, 1991 in the BBC's 'Everyman' Series, and Jane Coles wrote a seventy-five minute radio play, first broadcast in BBC Radio 4's 'Saturday Playhouse' series on October 24, 1992. Translations of the book appeared in many languages. In 1996 Juliet Mabey of Oneworld Publications encouraged me to think about an enlarged and revised edition. Accordingly, I added a number of passages which had not been included in the original book, and I added two new chapters which had been written after August 1986. I also made an attempt in this new edition to avoid the use of the male pronoun to refer to the Divine Being, wherever this was consistent with the natural flow of the prose. The result is the present volume.

I was prompted to start collecting new material when I had a dream in which I was falling from a high tower and landing on the shore, crushed between the land and the sea, yet alive. This dream seemed to speak of my position on the frontier between sight and blindness. I was, of course, completely blind and yet I had not been blind from birth. My memories were those of a passage over the frontier. The awareness that I had passed over this frontier seemed to stimulate a more positive experience of blindness, in which I was able to explore in a more creative way the gifts of hearing and touch. I was able to distinguish more clearly the state of blindness as such and the experience of loss which was associated with leaving sight.

In the mean time, there had been an addition to the family. Joshua was born on July 6, 1988. At work, I had become a professor in 1989, and was appointed Dean of my faculty in 1990, a post I held for three and a half years. This experience of senior university management created further problems and, at the same time, gave me fresh insights into the meaning of blindness in a sighted world.

Blindness does not in principle lead to the fragmentation of life. The lives of blind people are more or less as integrated as the lives of sighted people. It is true that we tend to think of sighted people as having something which blind people lack, and in that sense blindness is considered to be a deficiency. Certainly, when sight is lost it is almost always experienced as a terrible deprivation, and the loss is inevitably followed by a period of grieving. The change from living as a sighted person to living as a blind person is profound. Nevertheless, the life of a person who is blind is experienced as a whole. Losing one's sight is not quite like losing a limb. The blind person does not always remain conscious of something missing. The personality regroups; there is a process of healing and reintegration which leaves the life of the blind person complete and entire although smaller than it was before. One should not think of the life of the blind person as a cake which has had a slice cut out of it. Rather, it is like a smaller cake. It is experienced as being intact, although the scope of activity has in many ways become smaller.

The experience of reintegration, however, takes time. How much time it takes will depend upon the age when blindness occurred, and many other factors of environment and personality. Interpretation takes time. This process of reinterpretation is piecemeal; sometimes there are moments of dawning realization; often there are long periods of apparent stagnation. Sometimes the wound of the original loss seems never to heal. At other times one feels that the terrible gift has been received and assimilated.

My own attempt to interpret blindness passed through a number of stages. First I believed that blindness was when you couldn't see because something had gone wrong with your eyes. Then I understood that blindness was a deprivation of knowledge for which alternative sources and kinds of knowledge would compensate. Gradually I came to see that blindness is a whole-body condition. It is not simply that your eyes have ceased to function; your whole body undergoes a profound transformation in its relationship to the world. Finally, I came to believe that blindness is a world-creating condition. Blind people really do live in a different world. This world is part of a larger world, the world of sighted people.

The management of the relationship of the little world to the great world presents complex problems. How can the little world learn to live with the big world without manipulating it? How can the big world learn to live with the little world without patronizing it? Perhaps there are secrets about the relationship between the powerful and the less powerful which we could learn from these problems.

If blindness creates a new world, then those who live in that world have a new consciousness. Entry into this consciousness, for those who lose sight, is experienced as a fall. At first, the fall is out of consciousness, into the dreaming life, into the darkness. Later on, in my own case at any rate, the fall was discovered not to be out of consciousness but into it. A new consciousness was born. I can only describe that consciousness and the way to it through the presentation of a series of fragments. The thing itself is not fragmented but the path to it is experienced fragmentarily.

In this book I have gathered together a number of aspects of the life of this particular blind person so as to form a sort of mosaic which seeks to interpret the blind condition. The strands which are drawn upon are varied. They include the world of dreams, since it is through the dreaming life that the changes in the relationship between consciousness and unconsciousness are first realized. Next, there is a strand of human relationships, since it is in the interaction with others that we know ourselves. Some of these interactions are with friends and colleagues, but the most significant ones are with children, and especially with my own children. This is partly because I happen to see a good deal of my own children and have the opportunity to observe their reactions to living with a blind adult. There is more to it than that. In order to understand blindness one must study the minute particular. It is in the observation of tiny detail that I have come to understand the nature of blindness, and as I have observed my children's gradual growth in understanding, I myself have grown in understanding. Watching the interpretations of children has been a vital factor in forging my own interpretations.

A third strand is composed of experiences of the natural world. It is in the presence of the wind, of the rustling leaves of trees, in meditating upon the inexhaustible beauty of rain, in being awe-struck and terrified by the tumult of the waves on the seashore that I have built up bit by bit the world of blindness. At first it seemed as if thunderstorms without any experience of the flashes of lightning could not possibly be as exciting. This was a deficiency-interpretation. As time went by, thunderstorms became not less exciting than before but more so. What the thunder said was heard and interpreted in a new way from the state of blindness.

Finally, a vital strand consisted of philosophical, theological and spiritual meditations. I am deeply grateful to my parents, both of whom have now gone on ahead, for passing on to me the treasures of the biblical traditions. In the Christian faith as created and continuously renewed by the Bible, I have found a storehouse of imagery which was reactivated and reappropriated in the condition of blindness. I found that there was no better way to symbolize my life-experiences than through this tradition. It not only inspired from the past; it drew one, like a magnet, from the future of unrealized worlds.

Philosophical and phenomenological analysis also occupied a crucial part in my reinterpretation of blindness. Attention to minute detail requires a corresponding reflection, an analysis of thought, emotion and sensation such that understanding can lay the foundations of a new imaginative response. This process of bringing together philosophical scrutiny and theological inspiration is an important part of my experience of grace. The grace is found in the astonishing powers of the human spirit for healing and rebirth. Even more, the grace lies in that gracious reality which confronts the human spirit, which broods over the abyss and stirs it to life. This is part of what I understand by the Holy Spirit of God. I offer this book in gratitude and worship to the One who is the God of blindness, and who beyond blindness and sight is the God of all worlds.

These fragments could not have been gathered and assembled without the assistance of many people. I am grateful to the friends, both sighted and blind, with whom I have discussed these questions. I am particularly grateful to Helen Joinson who has shown such remarkable skill and patience in preparing most of the manuscript of this new edition. Finally, I owe a very special debt of gratitude to Marilyn and to my children. Their robust realism and sense of humour has often prevented me from taking myself and blindness too seriously. Their solidarity with me has enabled me to go on believing that sighted and blind people may still inhabit one world. They, and Marilyn above all, have enabled me to realize in a different and special way the nature of God's grace.

To the Blind Reader

Blind people differ from each other as much as sighted people do. I do not claim to speak for you, but only for myself. You do not need to know what blindness is like, because you are blind. Perhaps you are reading this book in order to discover companionship with someone else who has passed your way. I hope you find it here.

John M. Hull
April 1997

Introduction

I was born on 22 April 1935 in Corryong, a town in north-eastern Victoria. My father was the Methodist minister in nearby Cudgewa. He had emigrated from England to Australia as a lad in 1915 and after a series of jobs in farms and factories trained as an engine driver. He drove traction engines, agricultural machinery, worked on refrigeration plants and irrigation schemes, and was then drawn into the timber industry. He worked in sawmills and as a winch driver on various logging stations, mostly in the forests of eastern and southern Victoria. He has told the story of these colourful years in his autobiography *Yarns of Cowra Jack* which was published by the Joint Board of Christian Education in Melbourne, 1984.

It was while he was working in a remote logging camp in the Beenak area of the Dandenong Hills that he met Madge Huttley, the only teacher in the tiny local school. She was an enthusiastic Christian and was a major influence in Jack's conversion to Christianity which took place in 1927. He trained for the Methodist ministry in Queen's College, Melbourne, and Cudgewa was his first appointment.

My mother had been brought up in Stawell, a country town in north-western Victoria close to the beautiful Grampian mountain ranges. The Huttleys had emigrated from England in the 1870s, and Madge's father was the owner/operator of the first garage in Stawell. Madge trained as a primary teacher in Melbourne before taking up her first appointment in Beenak.

I was the second child of the marriage, my sister Alison having been born in 1933. Within a few days of birth my skin erupted in sores. This was the start of the condition which plagued me for the first half of my life. It may have been an allergic condition, perhaps associated with the asthma and the congenital cataracts in a syndrome which was not identified until many years later. Whatever the cause, the results were dramatic, and although as a child one accepts everything as being natural without question, this aspect of my childhood and youth has left a deep

1

impression upon me. My childhood memories are of bandages and ointments, of shirt sleeves worn thin and torn with scratching, of pushing myself around as a small child on a tricycle, being unable to straighten my legs enough to walk comfortably, of puzzled teachers asking me why my fingernails were so worn and polished, and of my mother's caring love. Her firm hands, her endless patience and the combination of strength and intimacy which she conveyed to me left permanent influences.

Cudgewa, not far from the sources of the river Murray and Australia's highest peak, Mount Kosciusko, is in an area of great natural beauty, but this made no impression on me until I came back more than twenty years later, for within two years my father had been posted to the other side of the state, to Red Cliffs, a town on the Murray River not far from Mildura. The vineyards were irrigated from the waters of the Murray. My first childhood memories come from those years. Food was kept cool in the icebox, and I can still remember the man from the ice cart bringing in the huge block of ice wrapped in hessian which he would chip with a pick to make it fit. Alison and I would grab the sharp fragments of ice and run out into the furrows between the grapevines next to the house. I can remember the salty quality of the sharp ice, the sweet green grapes and the hot, dry crumbly soil.

Under the itinerant arrangements usual for the Methodist ministry in those days, my father was again moved after three years, this time to Tasmania. It was late in 1939 or early 1940, and on the deck of the ship which took us from the mainland there was an anti-aircraft gun. When the crew removed the camouflage for the daily practice they were watched by an admiring crowd of small children, including me and my younger brother Keith, born in Red Cliffs.

During these years of the Second World War we lived in Wynyard, on the northern coast. There was a fear that the Japanese would bomb Melbourne guided by the lights of the northern Tasmanian coast, or might even attempt a landing prior to attacking the mainland. A zigzag trench was dug in the school yard, and every day we were drilled in snatching our tin helmets and gas masks while we ran to the shelter of the trench. In the evenings we children would sit on the front fence and watch the searchlights play in the sky. Holidays were taken every summer at Boat Harbour, on the coast not far away. Here I first learned to love the sea, the excitement and danger of the tides and the wonder of the life in the rock pools. While we lived in Wynyard, our family was completed by the birth of Janice.

When the war in the Pacific ended, in 1945, I was in the children's ward of Prince Henry's Hospital in Melbourne, because of the severity

2

of my eczema. The firework display along the banks of the Yarra was clearly visible from the tenth floor of the hospital, and the voice of General McArthur announcing the end of the war was broadcast through the wards. The family had moved back to Victoria, and my father was now posted in Charlton, a small town on the Avoca River in the north-western part of the state. This was wheat-growing country, and we boys played cowboys and indians on the huge stacks of bags of wheat, piled up beside the railway line and in the warehouses. On my way to school I had to cross the river on a footbridge. One year the river flooded and the bridge was impassable. It was very exciting watching the water come higher and higher each day and then the patterns of deep cracks in the drying mud under the fierce sunshine. Several times there were quite severe dust storms. The sky would grow red and ominous and we would all be sent home from school. I felt my way along the front fence to find the gate, hardly being able to open my eyes because of the fierce burning dust.

I missed a year from school because of my poor health, and spent this time in the correspondence school run by the State Education Department. I loved this, and waited eagerly for the weekly packet of booklets and work cards with a personal letter from my teacher whom I had never met. There followed two years in the Charlton Higher Elementary School before we moved sixty miles south to Eaglehawk, near the city of Bendigo. Keith and I travelled three miles to school on the tram or rode our bikes. Eaglehawk and Bendigo were situated on the old Victorian goldfields and the tall derricks above the mine workings were part of the skyline. In the bush there were tunnels and mineshafts, ideal for adventure.

My father had a large circuit consisting of three town churches, each with a full programme of activities, and three small country churches. Life in the churches was busy and exciting. On Sunday we began with Christian Endeavour classes for young people, followed by morning service at one church, then afternoon Sunday School at a different church (children of the manse had to be spread fairly around the churches), then a youth tea and visiting speaker followed by the evening service. After this, all the young people would crowd into somebody's home to sing Wesley's hymns and eat cake for another hour. The Sunday School anniversaries were something else. The trumpets and trombones would arrive, huge platforms would be erected in the church or Sunday School building, and we would rehearse all kinds of singing, speaking and dramatic performances. Concerts, barbecues and midnight hikes filled our adolescent lives. It was in the church that we were taught how

3

to study, to debate, to chair public meetings, to publish newspapers, to find our way around the bush and to sing. At the age of fourteen I began to experience Christian faith in a fresh and vivid way when a group of young men training for the Methodist ministry at my father's old college in Melbourne, Queen's, conducted a mission in the central Bendigo church, Forest Street. This marked the beginning of ten years of adolescent religious and emotional intensity, years from which I emerged to find myself studying theology in Cambridge, England.

It was sometime earlier, perhaps when I was thirteen, that I remarked as I came in for breakfast that it was a very misty morning. My surprised mother contradicted me, and then remembering that I had been complaining of not being able to see the board at school, took me into Bendigo to see my first eye specialist. It was to be thirty-eight years later before the last eye specialist signed me off.

Cataract was diagnosed and I lost the sight of one eye. After several months, the sight in the second eye began to deteriorate, and within a few months I could see nothing but a dense white fog. I was reading a novel about the Wild West, and was in a hurry to finish it, rather annoyed at the interruption. A particularly nasty skin infection which covered my face and neck made surgery impossible and I spent several weeks in hospital just waiting. Finally the lenses were pierced so that the cataracts could gradually dissolve. This 'needling' operation is no longer carried out, because it has been found that the vitreous jelly tends to move forward to cause detachment of the retina. My case, perhaps, played a small part in that discovery. Finally, the bandages were taken off and I was fitted with glasses. The heavy lenses restored the world to me and I can remember with delight the vivid outlines of shapes and colours. I gasped, and both the consultant and my father laughed with delight.

Three or four years later I had my first experience of the characteristic dark, disc-shaped area, edged with a flicker of light when I moved my eye rapidly, a symptom which I learned to associate with detached retina. I was to spend many years watching the progress of these dark shadows, measuring them carefully on the wall to mark out the speed of their advance, trying to explain their exact appearance and position to sceptical ophthalmologists, and knowing that when the disc passed over the central point of vision I would not be able to read. The first time this happened, however, I was not aware of its significance, and although I kept careful diagrams of the field of vision I am not sure that I told my parents. This was in the right eye, and according to my records the disc passed right over, light appeared on the other side, and sight was fully restored. At that time, I knew nothing about detached retinas. Some doctors have said that they could detect signs of this earlier detachment; in any case, it was of no significance. I was seventeen when the black disc appeared in the left eye. We were now living in Melbourne and I was taken to one of the leading hospitals. No diagnosis was made and the black disc engulfed the vision of the left eye. For some time, I saw as through a deep green jelly, and then there was a haemorrhage and light faded. With the carefree nature of youth, I was undismayed. I still had my right eye which somehow seemed to have fixed itself up.

For my sixth-form studies I attended Melbourne High School for Boys. The move from a small provincial high school to one of the leading schools in the state capital was very exciting, and for the first time I really enjoyed school. In history, English literature and geography, we were made to think about reasons and causes, and I began to understand the nature of evidence. Already a qualified and experienced Methodist local preacher, I soon found friends and common enterprises. In 1953 I matriculated to the University of Melbourne and decided to take an ordinary General Arts degree. The thought of joining one of the Honours Schools did not occur to me – I was destined for the Methodist ministry and was looking for a broad education which would prepare me for study at Queen's College and then to follow my father's footsteps. Vacations were crowded with organizing holiday camps for children and beach missions; twice I travelled inter-state on student committees and each time returned home early with asthma.

Just before the end of my first year, the now familiar dark disc reappeared in my right eye. This time diagnosis and surgery were swift. I spent several weeks in hospital, my head resting on a padded ring to reduce movement. I taught myself braille and read the Psalms and parts of St Mark's Gospel. I had only been recuperating for a few days at home, and had just been examined for new glasses when the thing happened again. Once more I was lying on my back in the darkness reading braille and wondering about the future. Strangely enough, it still made little impact on me. This time the operation was more successful and I finished my degree.

Finding that the government scholarship I had received could cover a teacher training course, I decided this would be a useful adjunct to the ministry and so spent a further year in the University Faculty of Education taking the Diploma in Education (the initial teacher training qualification) specializing in religious education. Since this was not taught in the state schools, the independent sector beckoned me and I was appointed to the staff of Caulfield Church of England Boys' Grammar School in Melbourne.

I spent nearly three happy years on the staff at Caulfield. I taught English, History, Social Studies and Religious Education, did some coaching of younger boys in cricket and Australian rules football and was in charge of the junior boarding house of about thirty youngsters aged 8–11. Twice a week after school I travelled back to the University to attend lectures in the philosophy and psychology of education as part of my B.Ed. degree. In 1958 I began thinking seriously about the future. The Methodist ministry was still my goal but the prospect of a further three years of study in Melbourne did not appeal. I wanted now to study theology in one of the leading European or North American universities. I was offered a place at Cambridge through Fitzwilliam House (now Fitzwilliam College). Accommodation in Wesley House was limited and I was advised to apply to Cheshunt College, which was a Congregationalist theological college although the principal at the time was a Methodist. Early in August of 1959 I set sail on the SS *Strathmore*.

In London I was met by Mary, my father's younger sister. She was a children's social worker with Doctor Barnardo's Homes in Devon and had come from Exeter to meet me. We had a marvellous time looking at all the great sights of London, familiar to me from the Monopoly board, and then I travelled by train to Cambridge.

The three years which followed were amongst the most formative of my life. I made friends with fellow students from many parts of the world, some of whom have remained friends ever since. I bought a motor scooter and travelled all over England, even taking the machine to France and Switzerland. The sight in my right eye was excellent, although I had to be careful with things on my left, and my night vision was poor. I learned to love the sights and sounds of Cambridge, punting on the Cam, toasting buns over coal fires on winter afternoons, the bookshops, the parties and the music. Above all, I learned to love the University Library. Following a trail of ideas across the centuries and from one wing of the library to another engrossed and delighted me. In tutorials for the first time in my life, I found myself alone with someone whose job it was to probe my thinking.

For two years I read Part II of the Theological Tripos and stayed on for a year to read Part III, specializing in New Testament Studies. In my third year I was elected Chair of the Junior Common Room, while vacations were spent hitchhiking throughout Europe and the Middle East. Passing through a crisis of faith, I found I could not conscientiously enter the ministry, and I decided to stay on in England and resume my work as a teacher. I married one of my fellow students from Cheshunt College and we moved to south London.

After four happy years teaching in Selhurst Boys' School in Croydon I was appointed lecturer in Divinity in Westhill College of Education in Birmingham. I taught New Testament studies, including Greek, Modern Theological Thought, and the Theory of Religious Education. I trained religious education teachers in primary and secondary schools and continued to teach every week in a nearby boys' school. I began to write, and in 1967 my first publication, a short article on teacher training, appeared in an educational journal. Birmingham had been one of the centres of the religious education revival of the 1960s; Ronald Goldman, Kenneth Hyde, Edwin Cox and many other well-known names were in the area. F. H. Hilliard, who had been Reader in Religious Education in the University of London Institute of Education, moved to Birmingham University to take up a Chair in Education, and Edwin Cox whose *Changing Aims in Religious Education* had been published in 1966, took his place in London. I moved from Westhill to the University to occupy the lectureship left vacant by Edwin. I was now able to specialize in the theory and practice of religious education, since my main responsibility was the training of theology graduates as secondary religious education specialist teachers. I also taught a post-experience course in the psychology of religious development.

In 1968 the student movement was at its height, and Birmingham was no exception. During my first term the students occupied Great Hall and the administrative block, and the whole campus was in a state of excitement. I was elected staff representative on to the Board of Education and from there to the University Senate, Council and Court, and spent six years in the middle 1970s on the Academic Executive Committee of Senate.

Birmingham was a fascinating city for my work. Cambridge was so beautiful, and London so large, but in Birmingham I learned to know and love the heart of England. Here there was no cushioning against public events, and the link between public and private was obvious. If there was industrial unrest, if the price of petrol went up, if there were problems in the high-rise flats or with the water supply, it was talked about in the schools and the markets, and its impact was immediate. Here I learned to appreciate Judaism, Hinduism, the Sikh faith and Islam. Here, in one of the great industrial, multi-cultural cities of Western Europe, religious education had a vital part to play.

I had been in my new post less than two years when the almost forgotten dark shadow made its reappearance. I reported the problem to a rather incredulous GP, who examined me carefully, assured me he could see nothing and dismissed me. After several insistent phone calls, he agreed to get me an appointment at the local eye clinic. Here the problem was quickly diagnosed and I underwent surgery in the Birmingham and Midland Eye Hospital. The treatment was expert and the result highly successful. The sight of my right eye was restored virtually intact and I was presented to one of the meetings of the West Midlands Ophthalmological Society. Within a few months, however, the problem had returned.

This time diagnosis was more difficult. Week after week passed, and the consultant refused to see me, while house doctors and students assured me there was nothing wrong. Every week I marked out on the wall of my office the progress of the black disc. Only after a letter of protest sent by recorded delivery to his private address was I admitted into the presence of the consultant. After a long examination he told me that immediate surgery would be necessary. I assured him that I had complete confidence in his skill but he insisted on passing me to a colleague. The next operation was done with great skill, I believe, but by now the eye was battered and scarred. In 1970 I began a decade of failing vision.

In 1973 my daughter Imogen Mary was born, but in spring of 1979, after more than two years of informal separation, my wife and I agreed on a divorce.

My New Testament researches in the Universities of London and Birmingham were complete by 1970, but the preparation of the 1974 publication did present some problems, so much of the work being in ancient and foreign languages. Although I hoped that my sight would not continue to deteriorate, I knew it would be foolish to put out hostages to fortune. I could get people to read books in English to me, but it would be more difficult finding people to read Greek and Aramaic. I was never much good at languages anyway, and found the gradual move to philosophy, theology and the social sciences very much to my liking. I had begun to teach an M.Ed. course in the Theology of Education, and this occupied me intellectually, while frequent lecturing visits to various countries brought an expanding group of colleagues and a deeper understanding of the relationship between religious education and modern culture.

I had begun reading with a magnifying glass in 1973 or thereabouts and in 1977 I finished *Shardik* by Richard Adams, having decided that this would be the last novel I would read with my eyes. I thought of the time thirty years earlier when I had hurried to finish that Western novel as the cataracts grew. From now on I must use my remaining sight to read for my work. There was no longer spare sight for unnecessary reading. The magnifying glasses grew larger and heavier. I held them in my hands, mounted them on my desk, and fixed them to my glasses. My desk was a battery of lamps and bookstands. Recording what I had read became an increasing problem. I wrote with thicker and thicker felt-tipped pens, finally having only a dozen or so words on a sheet, which I read with the aid of magnifying glasses. On 1 November 1979 I remarried. Within less than a year our first child was born, and I had registered blind. In September of 1980 I returned to my office from the Eye Hospital and the Maternity Hospital, a patient in the former and a visitor to the latter, to face a curious situation. Term was due to begin in less than a month, and the walls of my room were covered with files of notes representing years of work, all of which was now inaccessible.

The solving of these problems occupied the years 1980 to 1983, and might be the theme of a book in itself. In 1983 the last light sensations faded and the dark discs had finally overwhelmed me. I had fought them bravely, as it seemed to me, for thirty-six years, but all to no avail. It was then I began to sink into the deep ocean, and finally learned how to touch the rock on the far side of despair.

1

Sinking

Summer 1983

Dreaming   *1 June 1983*

How long do you have to be blind before your dreams begin to lose colour? Do you go on dreaming in pictures for ever?

I have been a registered blind person for nearly three years. In the past few months, the final traces of light sensation have faded. Now I am totally blind. I cannot tell day from night. I can stare into the sun without seeing the faintest flicker of sunshine.

During this time, my dreams have continued to be pictorial. Indeed, dreams have become particularly enjoyable because of the colourful freedom which I experience when dreaming. Has blindness, then, made any impact upon my dreams at all?

About six months ago I had a dream in which my sight improved. I could see my son Thomas. There he was, a cheerful, cheeky, lively little boy of two and a half sitting on my knee.

My final eye operation took place on 1 August. Thomas was born on 22 August. When I cannot quite remember how long I have been blind, I ask myself how old Thomas is.

Being present at the birth was a frightening but wonderful experience. They turned on the microphone of the machine which monitored the heartbeat of the baby. I could hear it very clearly as I sat beside the bed. Marilyn and I had been married for a little less than a year. The baby's heartbeat was incredibly fast, coming in little waves of accelerations, in time with the contractions. A lot of the time I did not know what was happening. Marilyn was crying. The bed seemed to be surrounded by midwives and doctors. There were a few quiet moments and then a baby's cry.

For about eighteen months I continued to have some visual impression of him. Within a few feet, I could tell where he was lying, and what colour his clothes were. I could tell the broad outlines of his face, when he was yawning or waving. All of the finer details were lost, the little expressions around the eyes, the shades of emotion in the early stages. In the summer of 1981, on the beach in Wales, I used to tie a piece of string around his ankle, so that if he crawled more than a few feet away I would be able to find him again. When he could walk, I used to play with him on the steps of the University Library. I could let him off the reins, because even if he disappeared I could hear the sounds of his shoes as he ran across the stone landings on those quiet, Saturday mornings in the winter, when the campus was almost deserted. Sometimes I would run after him in panic, frightened that he might get to the edge of something before I could catch him. As he became more mobile, and my sight grew worse, these outings became increasingly difficult.

Dreaming of the White Cane   *3 June 1983*

About a week ago I dreamt that I was returning by rail to a town in Normandy. I had an appointment to meet Marilyn in a restaurant which we had visited on a trip to Normandy which we made a year or so before our wedding. I left the station, and paused to examine the map to see where the station was, only to realize that I had left my white cane on the train. What worried me was not so much how I would get around, but the fact that I had lost a piece of my property. I then found myself holding a long metal tube, the sort that is used to prop up a clothes line. I was using this to explore my path, and I noticed that the people in the area around the station were looking at me curiously.

This is the first time I have dreamt of myself as being a blind person. There are a lot of unresolved contradictions. It would be impossible for a blind person dependent upon a cane to forget to bring it with him. I wanted the independent freedom of movement which would make it possible for me to keep my rendezvous with Marilyn in the restaurant, but blindness would take this freedom away. So I had the white cane, yet I did not have it. I could not move without a sort of substitute for the cane, yet I could see the reactions of the people around me. I had lost something which I would need when I met Marilyn. Loss of the cane was not only the loss of my ability to find her, it was the loss of something deeper, potency, the ability to love her.

I began to carry a short, white cane early in 1980, mainly as a signal to traffic when I was crossing the road. When my sight got worse, I bought a slightly longer cane, and then a longer one still. Finally, I bought a full-length cane, five feet long, with a rounded crook on the handle. I never seemed to have the time for any mobility training, although occasionally I wondered if I was developing bad habits in my technique which could have been avoided with some formal instruction.

On the whole, my experience has been that, if I have a bad habit, it causes me some inconvenience or inefficiency in my movement, and is naturally corrected in the effort to move more freely. In other words, blindness itself imposes an iron law upon the user of the white cane. Lampposts, kerbs and stairways are the best teachers.

Nice Day? *5 June 1983*

Sometimes when I greet people by saying 'Nice day!' they remain unresponsive or even appear surprised. The idea of a nice day is largely visual. A nice day occurs when there is a clear, blue sky. The sun will be shining and it may be reasonably warm, although even a bright clear day in the middle of winter will be called a 'nice day although a bit nippy'. A sighted person would not call it a nice day, let alone a lovely day, if it were overcast.

For me, the wind has taken the place of the sun, and a nice day is a day when there is a mild breeze. This brings into life all the sounds in my environment. The leaves are rustling, bits of paper are blowing along the pavement, the walls and corners of the large buildings stand out under the impact of the wind, which I feel in my hair and on my face, in my clothes. A day on which it was merely warm would, I suppose, be quite a nice day but thunder makes it more exciting, because it suddenly gives a sense of space and distance. Thunder puts a roof over my head, a very high, vaulted ceiling of rumbling sound. I realize that I am in a big place, whereas before there was nothing there at all. The sighted person always has a roof overhead, in the form of the blue sky or the clouds, or the stars at night. The same is true for the blind person of the sound of the wind in the trees. It creates trees; one is surrounded by trees whereas before there was nothing.

The misunderstanding between me and the sighted arises when it is a mild day, even warm, with a light breeze but overcast. To the sighted, this would not be a nice day, because the sky is not blue.

I will have to make my comments about the weather more specific.

I must remember to say that it is nice and mild today, or that it is a pleasant breeze.

I Can Still Manage   *8 June 1983*

Last night I had a beautiful, refreshing dream, in which I was walking along a river valley. There were fine homes, holiday bungalows, built along the river bank. I was on a walking holiday. I experimented, looking this way and that, finding out if I had sufficient range of sight to take in the whole of the valley and the landscape. Although it was not perfect, I found that I could get a sufficient sense of the place to move freely and to enjoy the scenery. I was saying to myself, 'There you are, you see! In good light and in these conditions you can still manage fairly well.'

In 1976 and '77 I could still see well enough to enjoy going for long, solitary walks in the Worcestershire and Shropshire countryside. The Severn Valley was a favourite walk. I used to go by bus or rail. Getting on the right bus was a problem. I could go into the coach station in the city centre and find the exact bay for the bus I wanted, or I could stand at the bus stop near my home and stop every bus that came along, asking the driver if he was going my way. I tried to make out the numbers of the buses by using a little telescope, but often the bus was upon me before I could work it out. Reading the maps was still possible with magnifying glasses. I liked walking beside the river, because it was almost impossible to get lost, although it was necessary to pay fairly close attention to the ground immediately in front. I often used to say to myself, 'Provided it doesn't get any worse, I can still manage.'

I have been having that thought for at least ten years. I could still manage, provided it did not get any worse. Even after I was registered blind, I could work my way from the office to my home by following the bright, double yellow parking lines painted on the edges of the University roads.

I would still be all right, if it stayed like this. When it got worse, I could still get home at night by following the street lamps one by one. I felt like a sailor far out at sea on an inky, black night, with one star to guide me. When I reached the lamppost, I could dimly make out the next little light. I could still manage, provided it didn't get any worse.

My dreams seem to be lagging about six years behind reality.

Eye Contact   *19 June 1983*

The relationship between blind and sighted people can become rather serious. This is not only due to the fact that the blind person cannot see smiles and respond to them; it is related to the inability to reply to all the fleeting nuances of the face, and especially the eyes. Blind people also lose communication through general body language, since although they can speak using gestures they cannot receive the body language of other people. Most of the little moments of play are lost, winking, sticking out your tongue, exchanging mocking glances, raising the eyebrows and so on. Everything must be channelled through words or through touch. Words are often too abstract, touch is often too concrete. The subtlety of the intermediate area between these two extremes disappears. I must touch you, which may be too intimate, or I must speak to you, which may be too obvious. Similarly, I must be touched, or I must be spoken to. To articulate the fleeting, playful details of eye contact is very difficult, if not impossible. Speaking robs these little gestures and glances of their character by making them seem premeditated. Speaking is too deliberate.

Faces   *21 June 1983*

During the first couple of years of blindness, when I thought about the people I knew, they fell into two groups. There were those with faces, and those without faces. It was a bit like wandering round the National Portrait Gallery. Here are rows of portraits, but here is a blank. You can tell where it used to hang by the outline of the wallpaper, and beneath the space is a little label giving the name. Perhaps this portrait is on loan elsewhere, or perhaps it is being repaired.

The people I knew before I lost my sight have faces but the people I have met since then do not have faces. I used to find the contrast between the two groups of people disturbed me. I could not relate one set to the other set. I knew how I knew the first lot – by their faces. How could I ever feel that I really knew the second lot?

As time went by, the proportion of people with no faces increased. Whole rooms are now bare, and the portraits which remain are covered with dust. Is it possible that some day I will come to visit the gallery and find the door locked, with a notice which says, 'This exhibition is permanently closed'?

It is three years now since I have seen anybody. Strangely enough, I have fairly clear pictures of many people whom I have not met again during these three years, but the pictures of the people I meet every day are becoming blurred. Why should this be?

In the case of people I meet every day my relationship has continued beyond loss of sight, so my thoughts about these people are full of the latest developments in our relationships. These have partly covered the portrait, which has thus become less important. In the case of somebody I know quite well but have not seen for several years, nothing has happened to take the place of the portrait, and when I think of those people, it is the portrait which comes to mind.

It distressed me considerably when I realized that I was beginning to forget what Marilyn and Imogen looked like. I had wanted to defy blindness. I had sworn to myself that I would always carry their faces hidden in my heart, even if everything else in the gallery was stolen.

If I do want to recapture the face of someone very close to me, I do it through visualizing a particular photograph, an actual photograph that I can remember very clearly from my sighted days. When I try to conjure up the memory of a loved face, I cannot seem to capture it, but the straight edges of the photograph seem to fix the mobile features firmly in my mind, so that I can imagine myself gazing at the image. Some people tell me that this is a happy situation. I will always remember Marilyn as being young. She need never be troubled by the thought that I will see her getting older. I am not so sure about this, since I find it hard to believe that ignorance can ever be better than knowledge.

The difference between those who have faces and those who do not becomes more poignant when I think of my own children. I have a lot of visual memories of Imogen, now aged ten, mostly based on photographs, but with the occasional vivid life situation thrown in. I have only a few rather vague impressions of the face of Thomas, now nearly three, which are based upon the first six or nine months of his life, while I still had a little residual vision. Of Elizabeth, now sixteen months, I have no visual images at all. The place on the wall which should carry her portrait is completely blank.

What difference does it make? I am not aware of any difference in my present relationships with these three children which could be affected in any way by the fact that they stand in different relationships to my blindness. They are all alike now.

Does It Matter What People Look Like?   *23 June 1983*

About a year after I was registered blind, I began to have such strong images of what people's faces looked like that they were almost like hallucinations. This went on for six or twelve months. I would be sitting in a room with someone, my face pointed towards my companion, listening to him or her. Suddenly, such a vivid picture would flash before my mind that it was like looking at a television set. Ah, I would think, there he is, with his glasses and his little beard, his wavy hair and his blue, pin-striped suit, white collar and blue tie. There are his polished shoes and his briefcase, standing neatly beside his chair. Now this image would fade and in its place another one would be projected. My companion was now fat and perspiring with receding hair. He had a red necktie and waistcoat, and a couple of his teeth were missing. This in turn would fade.

Sometimes I would become so absorbed in gazing upon these images, which seemed to come and go without any intention on my part, that I would entirely lose the thread of what was being said to me. I would come back with a shock, realizing that there was nothing to indicate which of these images was closer to reality. There was simply nothing there at all. The voice would return, and I would feel as if I had dropped off to sleep for a few minutes in front of the radio.

Several times in my life I have been temporarily without sight, often in eye hospitals. I have had this strange experience of getting to know the nurses through their voices and inevitably forming some mental image of them, only to find when sight returned that I was completely wrong. So I have good reason to believe that the images I have formed of the people whom I have met as a blind person are probably quite false. Moreover, I shall never have the opportunity of correcting them by discovering the truth for myself. Gradually, however, this tendency to project images is fading.

One of the results of not knowing what people look like is that the element of anticipation in a new relationship is diminished. When a sighted person makes a new acquaintance, sight alone enables him or her to form certain impressions and to get ready to meet a certain kind of person. The new acquaintance may strike one as being wise, friendly, remote, dignified, bewildered, and so on. The blind person, on the other hand, does not know what he or she is meeting. To say that this removes the possibility of facile first impressions is itself facile. The first impressions which the blind person does receive of a new acquaintance, of the voice, the touch of the hand and so on, may be equally misleading, and if one followed the strange logic which tells us it is better to be without any information which might mislead us, we could conclude that we would be better off with no information at all. We are constantly forming hypotheses about a new acquaintance, not only during the first few moments of the encounter but throughout the years of that relationship.

The blind person simply has a lot less information to go on when forming these hypotheses. One of the results is that it takes a blind person longer to get to know somebody. That, at any rate, is my experience, but perhaps I am not a very skilful blind person.

The fact that the blind person has less information would seem to suggest that his or her hypothesis about a new person ought to be more vulnerable. Although spared misleading visual impressions, a blind person is having to make do with fewer facts. Whether my first impressions of people are less reliable now than when I was sighted, I am unsure. I often interview candidates for University entrance with one or two colleagues. After the interview, we compare notes. I am relieved and a little surprised to find that my opinion of the candidate seemed to be no less accurate, or that I have picked up similar impressions. The sighted interviewers can add certain details. They can remark that the candidate had shifty eyes or was of untidy appearance. These almost always turn out to be consistent with various impressions of character or personality which I had formed solely from listening to the candidate speak.

Another strange feature of not knowing what people look like is the effect this has upon reported speech. When I am describing an encounter with someone, I may want to say, 'He looked blankly at me.' I feel a little sensitive about this, because I cannot help thinking that the sighted person to whom I am talking would know that I could not possibly know how my friend looked at me. To say, 'He responded in a blank manner' is absurd and pedantic. I am trying to suggest the pause which I noticed before my friend replied: the sense that I had that he was taken aback, was briefly at a loss for words, did not quite know what to say. There actually was a brief blank in the conversation. To say, 'He paused before replying and seemed to be at a loss' would be perfectly accurate, but to use the brief, concrete idiom of sighted exchange is so natural and vivid. What am I to do?

Another result of all this is that the face no longer has the central place for me which it has in normal human relationships. The face is merely the place from which the voice comes. I look towards the face with conscious effort, for there is no real reason why I should do so. I can often tell when people are looking at me, because their voices sound different if projected directly at me, and I am often able to glance at someone in a group when he or she has glanced at me and spoken. I do this, however, purely for effect, to show that I am listening. I no longer have any natural sense of needing to be face to face.

Sometimes I ask one of my sighted friends to give me a quick impression of what somebody else looks like. I am often interested in a sort of thumb-nail sketch of a new acquaintance. This is particularly true if my new acquaintance is a woman. What colour is her hair? What is she wearing? Is she pretty? Sometimes I long to know. I remain, after all, a man, reared in a certain sighted culture, conditioned to certain male expectations. Perhaps I should change, and be less influenced in my judgement of women by my male conditioning, but it is painful to have this change forced upon me by mere blindness.

It makes a difference to the way I feel about a new female acquaintance if a colleague, having caught sight of her, remarks on her beauty or her plainness. There is a double irrationality in this. In the first place, my feelings should not be so dependent upon a woman's appearance. I know that, and I apologize. But I still feel it. The second thing is that it is surely a deplorable lack of independence on my part to be so affected by a criterion which can be of no significance to me.

What can it matter to me what sighted men think of women, when I, as a blind man, must judge women by quite different means. Yet I do care what sighted men think, and I do not seem able to throw off this prejudice.

The crucial thing in any new acquaintance is the sound of the voice. I am continuing to learn more and more about the amazing power of the human voice to reveal the person. With the people I know very well, I find that all of the emotion which would normally be expressed in the face is there in the voice: the tiredness, the anxiety, the suppressed excitement and so on. My impressions based on the voice seem to be just as accurate as those of sighted people. There is the disadvantage, however, that my friend must speak. If I were sighted, I would have access to a certain privacy, I would catch an unintended communication through the fleeting expressions of the face, especially the lips and the eyes. As a blind person, I do have access to unintended nuances of the voice, and can often hear many things which the speaker may not know are there, but it is always in the context of something which was intended, namely, the speaking itself. So I am more dependent upon other people revealing themselves to me.

The capacity of the voice to reveal the self is truly amazing. Is the voice intelligent? Is it colourful? Is there light and shade? Is there melody, humour, gracefulness, accuracy? Is it gentle, amusing and varied? On the other hand, is the voice lazy? Is it sloppy and careless? Is it flat, drab and monotonous? Is the range of vocabulary poor and used without precision and sensitivity? These are the things which matter to me now.

Increasingly, I am no longer even trying to imagine what people look like. My knowledge of you is based upon what we have been through together, not on what you look like.

There is a further development. Not only do I not know or care what you look like (although I still have a few qualms and doubts in the case of women), I am beginning to lose the category itself. I am finding it more and more difficult to realize that people look like anything, to put any meaning into the idea that they have an appearance. In recent weeks I find myself practising the thought that people do have an appearance. I am experimenting, by rehearsing in my mind the different kinds of appearance which somebody might have. This is quite different from the vivid, compulsive projections which I had during that earlier period. I am now trying to remind myself that there is something about this person, something which means little or nothing to me, and to which I have no independent access, yet something which is as true about this person as anything else. This person looks like something. He or she does have what they call an 'appearance' of some kind.

What Do I Look Like?   *25 June 1983*

When I was about seventeen and lost the sight of my left eye I can remember gazing at my left shoulder and thinking, 'Well, that's the last time I'll see you without looking in a mirror!' To lose the shoulder is one thing, but to lose one's own face poses a new problem. I find that I am trying to recall old photographs of myself, just to remember what I look like. I discover with a shock that I cannot remember. Must I become a blank on the wall of my own gallery?

To what extent is loss of the image of the face connected with loss of the image of the self? Is this one of the reasons why I often feel I am a mere spirit, a ghost, a memory? Other people have become disembodied voices, speaking out of nowhere, going into nowhere. Am I not like this too, now that I have lost my body?

Darkness Within   *10 July 1983*

Many of those who have written about blindness are at great pains to deny that the experience is one of darkness. It is pointed out that blind people may have a certain amount of optical sensation, flashing lights and so on. Moreover, the visual field is characterized by a bluey-grey colour rather than pitch blackness. They comment critically on the names of many of the agencies and magazines which exist to help blind people, such as *Lighthouse for the Blind, The Torch Trust* and *The New Beacon*.

I am not sure if this rejection of darkness conveys a faithful description of blindness. It is true enough that the visual experience (if one can call it that) which blind people have is not of inky blackness but of a sort of greyness, sometimes pinky-grey or blue-grey, perhaps somewhat uneven, or speckled. Nevertheless, one is surely in darkness.

The degree to which I am actually conscious of this at any one time depends upon my awareness of being ignorant. When I am engaged in something which gives me a sense of intimate and accurate knowledge, like taking part in a discussion on a subject that I know a lot about, reading an interesting book or making love, the sense of darkness diminishes. In situations of uncertainty, when I become a little panicky through being asthmatic or losing my way, then I usually have a very strong, even claustrophobic sense of darkness. This seems worse if I am very hot, or very cold. I also feel plunged into darkness when I am emotionally involved in ignorance.

I watched my sixteen-month-old daughter Lizzie playing with her grandmother. Lizzie has learned to spin around like a top, making herself dizzy and falling over. Grandma was commenting on this with amusement and Lizzie was playing up to her and showing off her spinning skills. It occurred to me that if I had been there alone I would not have known that Lizzie was twirling round and round. Lizzie would not have been able to show off to me. When I knew of the play between Lizzie and her grandmother, I became aware of a sense of profound darkness. My head felt limp, as if I could not bother holding it upright. My head was nothing but a blob of blackness. Perhaps I could blow it away, or allow it to drop down onto my chest like a rotten apple.

For the sighted person, the interior is a lighted interior. Consciousness is always dominated by visual memories, impressions and knowledge, so that the shapes, sizes and movements of lighted reality always occupy the imagination and the memory, even when the eyes are closed. Internally as well as externally, there is light. For me, consciousness is an experience of internal darkness, in that it is no longer illuminated by colour, shape and movement. Most of the precision, complexity and detail of the actual world is lost as consciousness is occupied by things touched and heard. In moments of emotional anxiety, this becomes an awareness of ignorance, a consciousness of darkness. It is not just that one cannot see; one is plunged into darkness.

My darkness is, however, pierced by knowledge. When I am holding

Lizzie on my knee, bouncing her up and down, hearing her laugh, talking with her, knowing everything that is happening to her, I never have this sense of darkness. Even when I am gazing into her face I do not have it, provided I know what she is thinking and feeling, that is, I know the content of the relationship. Nor do I have this sense of darkness when I am in an environment which is richly stored with many tactile memories, such as the office and the desk at which I am now working. Every inch of my surroundings, every little object, every piece of paper, every corner or surface is immediately recognizable and is known by me. This could be called a sort of visualized space, since I know where the various things are set out on my desk, and the knowledge is spatial because the desk is spatial. It would probably be more accurate, however, to say that these tactile memories are cognitions, and that for the person who has had sight these clusters of cognitions have the emotional value of light. So for the once-sighted person, the surroundings are known in a way which is the emotional equivalent of visualization.

Touching   *12 July 1983*

It is amazing how touch brings things to life. Sounds are abstract, but touch puts body on things.

I may walk around a museum, and have a description of everything. Running my fingers over the edges of the display cases, putting my hand on the descriptive plaque even though I cannot read it, now and then extending a hand and touching a statue or a piece of machinery: these will be the memories which I will take home. The verbal description gives the context without which the tactile experiences would have little meaning, but it is touching which seems to earth the words.

In a cathedral, I have very little sense of the architecture as a whole. The windows, the tracery of the ceilings, the general proportion of the pillars, all this is lost. Only let me have a few minutes exploring with my fingers some of the intricate carvings on the screen, or to run the palms of my hands over the roughness of the stone, noticing the different textures and temperatures and something very vivid is regained. I must not be content merely to walk on the floors, but must stoop down and explore the tiles, or the rows of stone steps with my fingers. It is this which gives me a sense of real knowledge.

It is strange to find that sometimes the verbal description corresponds to what is felt, and sometimes it does not. Fingers, for example, simply do not reveal whatever it is that makes a human face ironic, stern or pretty.

Facial Vision   *14 July 1983*

I have had moments of this much-discussed blind experience ever since I lost the sight of my left eye. It took the form of a sudden, vivid awareness of an object on my blind side, within a few inches of my head. Stepping out to cross the road, I would recoil from something immediately on my left. Glancing around, there would be something like a parked van with a set of ladders extending from the roof, which I had not noticed.

I have since discovered that this phenomenon is now generally called 'echo location'. It was after the first few months of complete blindness that I became aware of it. As long as any sight at all remained, I was not aware of experiencing echo location. I first noticed that walking home over the campus in the quiet of the evening I had a sense of presence, which was the realization of an obstacle. I discovered that if I stopped when I had this sense, and waved my white cane around, I would make contact with a tree trunk. This would be no more than three, four or five feet from me. The awareness, whatever it was, did not seem to extend beyond this range, and sometimes the tree would be as close as two feet. It was through sensing these trees, and verifying their exact location with my stick, that I gradually realized that I was developing some strange kind of perception. I learned that I could actually count the number of these trees which I would pass along the road leading down to the University gates. The sense did not seem to work on thin objects like lampposts. It had to be something about as bulky as a tree trunk or a human body before I sensed it.

As the months go past, sensitivity seems to be increasing. I find now that I am quite often aware of approaching lampposts, although it is true that, if I am expecting one, it is easier to sense it. I do occasionally walk into lampposts which I have not detected at all. When I am aware of echo location, it is infallible, in the sense that I cannot remember having had the experience only to find that there was nothing there. Unfortunately, the experience itself does not always occur, so I can only use it as a sort of red light. I must stop when I sense something, but not sensing something does not mean that I can go ahead.

Not only have I become sensitive to thinner objects, but the range seems to have increased. When walking home, I used only to be able to detect parked cars by making contact with my cane. These days I almost never make contact with a parked car unexpectedly. Nearly always, I realize that there is an obstacle in my path before my stick strikes against it. This is in spite of the fact that I am now using the very long cane. I think the range for detecting parked cars must be approximately six to eight feet. Another feature of this experience is that it seems to be giving me a sort of generalized sense of the environment. There is one part of my route where I must step aside to avoid an upward flight of steps. I am expecting these, of course, since I come this way every day. Nevertheless, I am now aware of their approach, and not merely of the lower, closer steps, but of the whole massive object, looming up and somehow away from me. The phenomenon seems to be partly dependent on attention, since at home I can easily walk into the edge of doors, having had no warning of their proximity. Possibly in a house where sound is muffled by carpets and curtains, echoes would be less easily perceived?

The experience itself is quite extraordinary, and I cannot compare it with anything else I have ever known. It is like a sense of physical pressure. One wants to put up a hand to protect oneself, so intense is the awareness. One shrinks from whatever it is. It seems to be characterized by a certain stillness in the atmosphere. Where one should perceive the movement of air and a certain openness, somehow one becomes aware of a stillness, an intensity instead of an emptiness, a sense of vague solidity. The exact source of the sensation is difficult to locate. It seems to be the head, yet often it seems to extend to the shoulders and even the arms. Awareness is greater when the environment is less polluted by sound, and in the silence of my late evening walk home, I am most intensely aware of it. In a crowded noisy street, the experience is less noticeable, and if I am travelling on somebody's elbow, I never seem to notice the experience at all. Presumably, I just switch off whatever it is.

It is a sort of guidance system which comes into operation when absolutely necessary, and when the cues are somehow available, but it is not always easy to distinguish it from other experiences. When I come to the end of a block, I can often tell. Is this because of the movement of the air, the breeze which one often feels at the corner, or is it the reverse of the experience of presence? Have I, without realizing it, been aware of the presence of the walls and fences, suddenly encountering an absence when they end?

On one of my walks, I pass beside a five-foot-high fence made of vertical, metal bars. This gives way, at a certain point, to a solid brick wall. I find that if I pay attention I can tell when I have left the fence and am going along the wall. There is, somehow, a sense of a more massive presence.

I gather from conversations that this experience is essentially acoustic and is based upon awareness of echoes. This certainly fits in with my experience, but at the same time it is important to emphasize that one is not aware of listening. One is simply aware of becoming aware. The sense of pressure is upon the skin of the face, rather than upon or within the ears. That must be why the older name for the experience was 'facial vision'.

What Blindness Does to the Brain   *4 August 1983*

I have been reading an interesting book about conversion, called *Snapping: America's Epidemic of Sudden Personality Change*. The authors, Flo Conway and Jim Siegelman, suggest that the kind of intense conversion experience which is encouraged by some of the more extreme religious sects can be regarded as a response to a previous overload of information. People bewildered and confused by the complexity of life find a sudden and blissful release in the simplicity of adopting a single purpose under the authority of a single group or leader. The popular word for this kind of conversion is 'snapping'.

Explaining this idea, the authors described the brain as an organ for the processing of information. We know from many experiments that deprivation of information has a drastic effect. The brain seems to need information, almost as the lungs need air. The brain responds not only to the quantity of information received but to the channel of perception. Alterations both in the intensity of the information and in the channel can bring about changes in personality. The effects of solitary confinement, of silence or darkness can be understood in the light of information theory. The various meditation and concentration techniques employed by some totalitarian sects can also be understood in this way.

Does this approach help us to understand what blindness does to the brain? Conway and Siegelman point out that the vast majority of information which the brain receives comes through sight, for the normal person. May we thus understand blindness as a form of information loss, an acute form of cognitive deprivation? Snapping seems to take place when powerful patterns of information are suddenly imposed upon a brain previously patterned in a different way, and ready for sudden transformation because of stress or other crises. Blindness, however, does not seem to be associated with a sudden personality change, any more than would be expected by any other experience of loss or profound change. Similarly, loss of sight is not normally accompanied by the kind of sensations associated with the snapping experience – tingling of the skin, the feeling that running water is flowing over your body, and that cascades of light are pouring down from on high.

On the other hand, perhaps there are some similarities between blindness and snapping. Converts speak of dying and being reborn, and loss of sight is frequently experienced as the death of the old self. The drowsiness of which many newly blinded people complain, the dramatic increase in dreaming and the sense of boredom could all be regarded as reactions to information-loss. Loss of information is a factor in the problems of mobility and functioning in daily life which are an obvious part of the experience of going blind. This, however, would lead us to suppose that blindness is a mere inconvenience. It is annoying not to know many things – train timetables, my salary last month and where I left my coffee cup. The experience of recently blinded people, however, goes beyond feelings of inconvenience and annoyance. Blindness inflicts upon the brain a lack of information, which is in itself a cause of suffering. The brain pants to know, just as the lungs pant for air. The deterioration of the process of knowing is itself at stake, rather than the mere loss of particular items of useful knowledge.

'I See What You Mean'   *1 September 1983*

'Well, I'll see you around.'
   'Nice to see you again.'
   'I see what you mean.'
   When I use expressions like these, some of my sighted friends are surprised. They laugh, perhaps teasing me, and say, 'You don't really mean that, do you John?' I explain that, when I say I am pleased to see you, what I mean is that I am pleased to meet you, pleased to be with you, glad to be in your presence. I explain that this is surely what anybody, blind or sighted, would mean by that expression. In the same way, I explain, when I say that I see what you mean, what I mean is that I understand you. Your words make sense to me. This is what anybody must mean by that expression, since the meaning itself is invisible.

When you are blind you do become aware of how much of our language is dependent upon images drawn from sight. It is natural that sighted people also become sharply aware of this when talking with a blind person. 'What is your point of view?' 'Do you have any observations?' 'I just don't understand the way you look at this.' 'Now look here, my friend!' 'I've looked everywhere for it.' 'I'll see if I can help you.'

In expressions like these, attitudes, intentions, demands and references to knowledge and understanding are all suggested by the use of visual metaphors. There is an intimate connection between seeing and knowing. Blindness leads to ignorance.

Must disabled people refrain from using that part of the language which makes metaphorical use of the disability from which they suffer? How absurd this would be. It would impose a new, linguistic disability upon people already disabled. When somebody in a wheelchair says that she is thinking of standing for parliament, I don't draw attention to the disability by commenting wittily 'You mean you will go in your wheelchair to parliament'. If one of my friends remarks that she bumped into so and so the other day in the High Street, I do not, as a rule, guffaw and ask 'Did you hurt him?'

It is true, nevertheless, that beneath the little irritations of these exchanges between blind people and their sighted friends there lies a genuine problem. The whole structure of our ordinary, everyday conversation presupposes a sighted world. This can be easily noticed if you compare conversations on the radio with those on the television. So when the sighted person draws attention to a little oddity in the use of a visual metaphor by a blind person, beneath this lies a subtle shift in the whole character of communication between sighted and blind people. There is a language of blindness.

Rain   *9 September 1983*

This evening, at about nine o'clock, I was getting ready to leave the house. I opened the front door, and rain was falling. I stood for a few minutes, lost in the beauty of it. Rain has a way of bringing out the contours of everything; it throws a coloured blanket over previously invisible things; instead of an intermittent and thus fragmented world, the steadily falling rain creates continuity of acoustic experience.

I hear the rain pattering on the roof above me, dripping down the walls to my left and right, splashing from the drainpipe at ground level on my left, while further over to the left there is a lighter patch as the rain falls almost inaudibly upon a large leafy shrub. On the right, it is drumming, with a deeper, steadier sound upon the lawn. I can even make out the contours of the lawn, which rises to the right in a little hill. The sound of the rain is different and shapes out the curvature for me. Still further to the right, I hear the rain sounding upon the fence which divides our property from that next door. In front, the contours of the path and the steps are marked out, right down to the garden gate. Here the rain is striking the concrete, here it is splashing into the shallow pools which have already formed. Here and there is a light cascade as it drips from step to step. The sound on the path is quite different from the sound of the rain drumming into the lawn on the right, and this is different again from the blanketed, heavy, sodden feel of the large bush on the left. Further out, the sounds are less detailed. I can hear the rain falling on the road, and the swish of the cars that pass up and down. I can hear the rushing of the water in the flooded gutter on the edge of the road. The whole scene is much more differentiated than I have been able to describe, because everywhere are little breaks in the patterns, obstructions, projections, where some slight interruption or difference of texture or of echo gives an additional detail or dimension to the scene. Over the whole thing, like light falling upon a landscape is the gentle background patter gathered up into one continuous murmur of rain.

I think that this experience of opening the door on a rainy garden must be similar to that which a sighted person feels when opening the curtains and seeing the world outside. Usually, when I open my front door, there are various broken sounds spread across a nothingness. I know that when I take the next step I will encounter the path, and that to the right my shoe will meet the lawn. As I walk down the path, my head will be brushed by fronds of the overhanging shrub on the left and I will then come to the steps, the front gate, the footpath, the culvert and the road. I know all these things are there but I know them from memory. They give no immediate evidence of their presence, I know them in the form of prediction. They will be what I will be experiencing in the next few seconds. The rain presents the fullness of an entire situation all at once, not merely remembered, not in anticipation, but actually and now. The rain gives a sense of perspective and of the actual relationships of one part of the world to another.

If only rain could fall inside a room, it would help me to understand where things are in that room, to give a sense of being in the room, instead of just sitting on a chair.

This is an experience of great beauty. I feel as if the world, which is veiled until I touch it, has suddenly disclosed itself to me. I feel that the rain is gracious, that it has granted a gift to me, the gift of the world. I am no longer isolated, preoccupied with my thoughts, concentrating upon what I must do next. Instead of having to worry about where my body will be and what it will meet, I am presented with a totality, a world which speaks to me.

Have I grasped why it is so beautiful? When what there is to know is in itself varied, intricate and harmonious, then the knowledge of that reality shares the same characteristics. I am filled internally with a sense of variety, intricacy and harmony. The knowledge itself is beautiful, because the knowledge creates in me a mirror of what there is to know. As I listen to the rain, I am the image of the rain, and I am one with it.

Sinking   *16 September 1983*

I dreamt that we were on an ocean liner. We were struggling towards the stern of the ship. I was with someone, I could not tell who; it could have been Marilyn. We were fighting our way through bars, cocktail lounges, along little corridors, up and down flights of stairs, past cabins and finally emerged on the deck at the very stern. There we were, out in the open air, and we could see the great swell of the ocean. There were no waves, but a long steady swell of masses and masses of water, sky and wind. The ship was hurrying along, pushing its way through all this.

Somehow, we were transported over the stern of the ship and now I found myself with two women on another ship. I didn't know, or don't remember who the two women were, but there were three of us. This second ship was sinking. Or was it still the same ship? We were still in the stern, but now the deck was vertical, and the ship was sliding down. Perhaps three-quarters of the vessel was now beneath the water. We were clinging to the upper part of it. The other ship was going away, leaving us further and further behind. There we were, now clearly marooned on this second ship.

Now there came a feeling of the enormous weight of the huge bulk of the waterlogged vessel, a vision of it going down under the water, becoming lost in the deep-green murky depths, where it was getting darker, colder and more silent. There was no storm, it was not a wild sea. There was a vast, sullen swell and the weight of the ship's hull underneath us. Every time a great swell came along the vessel would become just a little more waterlogged, a little heavier, and would settle down a little further. Now we were more or less on eye-level with the swell, and it was a question of which surge would engulf us. A terrible sense of dread and hopelessness filled the dream.

My mind was full of the knowledge of that irresistible weight, dragging everything down and down, while the freedom and light and speed of the ship upon which we had been travelling was receding, always receding. The gap was widening all the time and one was left in the silence of the green sea while the weight was pulling one further and further down. I woke with a feeling of horror as if I had received a portent so ominous that it filled my whole life.

The ship that moves away with its light and speed is the world of the sighted. My family, my loved ones, and I are pushing our way through it. We are stranded, increasingly cut off. We are immobile, waterlogged. I am being dragged down and down into something unimaginable from which there will be no return. One world will disappear. The world into which I am being dragged with my loved ones will engulf us. There will be no return. Blindness is permanent and irreversible. I know now that my dreaming self is, after all, not deceived. My life is in crisis.

2

Into the Tunnel

Autumn 1983

Smiling   *17 September 1983*

Nearly every time I smile, I am conscious of it. I am aware of the muscular effort; not that my smiles have become forced, as if I were only pretending, but it has become a more or less conscious effort. Why is this? It must be because there is no reinforcement. There is no returning smile. I am no longer dazzled by a brilliant smile. I no longer find that the face of a stranger breaks into sudden beauty and friendliness. I never seem to get anything for my efforts. Most smiling is responsive. You smile spontaneously when you receive a smile. For me, it is like sending off dead letters. Have they been received or acknowledged? Was I even smiling in the right direction? In any case, how could my sighted friend make acknowledgement? You can smile with your voice, but you have to find something to say.

Because it has become irrelevant, I can feel myself stopping smiling. Well, I think I can feel this. I must ask someone close to me if it is true or not.

'Show Daddy'   *21 September 1983*

Thomas was three years old a month ago. He knows that he has to treat me differently. Ever since he was tiny I have trained him in the expression 'Show Daddy'. He knows that this does not mean the same as 'Give it to Daddy', which means 'surrender it up'. By contrast, 'Show Daddy' means 'put whatever you've got in your hand into my hand and you will get it straight back'. From the earliest days, I trained him, so that if I lightly tapped him on the back of the hand, he would immediately put into my hand what he was holding, and I would return it. If it was something which he should not have had, I would still return it to him immediately, and only after an interval would I begin on the 'give it to Daddy' line. We then developed this with books. I would say 'Is there a car?' and if he said that there was, I would say 'Show Daddy'. He would then take my outstretched finger and place it on the picture of the car.

Quite early on, he also learned an extension of this, whereby he was not using my finger only but my whole arm to guide me to something he wanted. If he wanted a toy from a high shelf, I would lift him up in my arms or on to my shoulders. He would then hold my arm, using it as a sort of instrument, and guide it towards the desired toy. So this was another version of 'Show Daddy'.

He also learned to say 'Look, Daddy!' He would then take my hand or finger and press it against whatever it was he wanted me to inspect. Thomas thus understands that I see with my fingers. He knows what braille is. He knows that my books are brailled, or that having a braille mark is a sign that it is my book. He learned to repeat after me, 'Daddy can't read this book because it is not brailled' and 'Daddy can read this because it is brailled'. He now makes these remarks about books quite spontaneously.

It is several months ago now that pointing to one of his own books he remarked 'Daddy can't read this' and then, pointing to the braille label in a picture book, 'Thomas can't read that'.

Earlier in the summer, he asked me, 'Daddy, did you come in like that?', jabbing in the air this way and that with his finger. I asked him what on earth he meant. 'Did you come in like that – jab, jab, – jab – with your stick?' I now realized that with his finger he was describing the movements of the white cane.

What I am not sure about, however, is whether all of this behaviour is associated with my sight, or whether it is merely special behaviour appropriate for Daddy. When he was a little more than twelve months old, he used to sit in his high chair, making funny faces first at one member of the family then another. He would turn from person to person to see what effect his funny faces had. Marilyn told me that he would turn his funny face on me, and after a few seconds would simply turn away again. Did he conclude from this experience that the reason his funny face had no effect upon me was that I could not see him? I doubt this very much. Marilyn says that even today in the context of normal family life he gives me just the same glances, looks, smiles and

31

other expressions as he does towards everyone else. On the other hand, a sighted adult would do this as well. One does not become poker-faced in one's conversation with a blind person just because he cannot see you. You do not stop smiling at a blind person just because he cannot see your smiles. Your smiles make you feel good.

Even if Thomas realized that I cannot see his funny faces, I am not sure that he would generalize this. He knows that I cannot read his books, cannot see the pictures, cannot do the jigsaws, but does he know that I cannot see him?

Ever since he was a small baby, long before he could walk, he has been picking things up for me. When he was on my knees, if I dropped something I would lower him to the carpet, he would pick it up, crawling around if necessary, and bring it back to me. He still does this. I say, 'Where are your socks?' He will pass them to me, even though they have been on the floor only six inches away. On the other hand, when I am travelling in the car with him, he will cry out 'Look Daddy!' about something which is outside the car. I must try reminding him that he cannot show me something which is outside the car.

Low Morale   *22 September 1983*

This month marks the third anniversary of my registration as a blind person. Total blindness has been much more recent, but so slow has been the loss of the last traces of light that it is not easy to remember the stages.

Two years ago, during our holiday in Brittany, I was still using a little telescope to pick out the shapes of buildings and scenery. Two years ago, although almost all my reading was done on cassette, I was still making notes in handwriting. This was getting bigger and bolder all the time, as I changed from thick biros to felt-tipped pens. In the end, I was only getting ten or fifteen words on a sheet of A4 paper, and reading these letters with a magnifying glass was becoming more and more laborious. In Brittany, we had a camp fire, and I could tell where it was. The glimmer of the flames was quite bright. I could not, however, go walking alone. I could not cross roads. I could not find shops, and I could not tell what was in shop windows. Sightseeing had become a bore, and I remember coming back from Brittany with the thought that I might just as well have been driving round the Birmingham Ring Road for all the impression I had gained of France.

When I walked home on wet nights, the street lamps threw beams of yellow light on the footpaths. I could just make out this track of light, and could use it to walk in a straight line. It is a real effort now to remember all this.

My morale is probably lower now than at any time during the past three years. At first, going blind was such a challenge. There were so many things to do, so many adaptations to be made. I think I must have adopted a fairly robust response to the problems, because I can remember thinking to myself, 'I am not interested in blindness. I am interested in my work. Your eyes are just a convenient visual aid, situated in your head. If they pack up, you just have to make do with alternatives.' During 1980, 1981 and perhaps the first part of the following year, there were also the fluctuations in my sight to keep me interested. Sometimes it seemed to be getting better, sometimes worse. There was always the hope of improvement. Even if there was deterioration, this was curious. As these hopes faded, and the deterioration seemed to become inexorable, I was kept busy thinking about new problems.

I have now reached the point where I do not suppose that my mobility skills will improve much more. My walk from home to the office will probably not present many more problems, nor will I walk it any faster. I do not suppose that my skills in authorship techniques and in using these tape recorders will get much better now. The major problems at work have been confronted and overcome as far as possible.

Now I have to face the thought that there is no escape. I will go on, just like this. My deterioration has levelled out. My sight cannot get any worse. I have nothing left to fear. There will be another twenty, maybe thirty, years like this.

Seeing with a Stick   *25 September 1983*

How strange it is for sighted people to recognize that there is a human being who is using a stick as an extension of his perception! It is not easy for sighted people to realize the implications of the fact that the blind person's perception of the world, sound apart, is confined to the reach of his body, and to any extension of his body which he can set up, such as a cane. This is illustrated, I think, by the great difficulty which most sighted people have in helping a lost blind person to reorientate himself. The indications of place which sighted people provide are usually too general, or they presuppose that the blind person has a greater knowledge of his environment than he may actually have.

It is so easy and normal for people to assume that your head is what you use to see with. If you met a creature from Mars, it would not take you long to work out that it was seeing you with a particular feeler, which was in your direction, or that it was seeing you through its bottom, which was always pointed towards you whichever way you moved. When sighted people approach a blind person, beginning with the natural expectation that they are dealing with a fellow creature, the implications of the fact that this person is actually 'seeing' through his white cane are difficult to absorb. Sometimes when I was being led by a sighted person, he or she would lift up my arm, so that my cane did not quite reach the ground. I have managed to avoid this problem by using a longer cane since December of 1982. It is more common for people to guide me by grabbing the cane itself, and pointing to things with it, tapping and saying 'There'.

People tend to stab at approaching steps with the white cane. I point out gently that, unless I myself am holding the cane, I cannot receive from it the information which I need. 'Please let go of the cane,' I say, 'just let me hold your arm.'

It is natural for people to regard the white cane as a sort of walking stick. It is looked upon as something which gives support. It is not immediately thought of as an instrument of sense perception, as a way of gathering information about the world.

'I Always Look After People Like You'   *26 September 1983*

Last night, walking home, I had just left the University gates and was about to round the corner into Bristol Road itself, when I was greeted by a man who spoke in a Middle Eastern accent.

'Stop,' he said. 'There is a car on the footpath.'

'Thank you,' I said. 'Is it parked there?'

'No, no,' he replied, 'there's been an accident. My brother is badly ill. Badly hurt. In his car.'

'And you,' I asked, 'are you hurt?'

'No,' said my friend. 'This thing has never happened to me because I always look after people like you.'

'Well,' I said, 'is your brother badly hurt?'

'No. He'll be all right. Let me take you across the road.'

'When did this happen?'

'Just now. Just now. I am thanking God that it's no worse. That I am all right. Now I will see you across the road.'

He not only took me to the pedestrian lights, he insisted on escorting me, carefully and gently, over the road itself to the far side. He deposited me firmly against the railings, wished me good luck and God's blessing and went back to join his shaken or injured brother in the car which had just mounted the footpath.

He seemed to have greeted my arrival, around the corner just at that moment, as a sort of signal from heaven. It was a warning to him. These things had never happened to him because he always looked after people like me. I was a providential note, sounding in his conscience. I appeared around the corner with my white cane, just as his brother's car was coming to rest on the pavement.

The Waterfall   6 October 1983

I dreamt that I was in a religious house, some kind of retreat centre. It was high in the mountains. Large windows opened upon many waterfalls, rivers and seas. We went even higher up, into a kind of elevated extension of the centre, emerging into a chapel. It was very lofty, very peaceful. It was beautifully laid out, equipped with study centres, little rooms for discussion groups and the chapel itself had a huge, plate-glass window which opened out upon a majestic waterfall. This towered over the whole place. Looking up, one could see the great bank of water shooting over from the top. The water was reddish brown, as if there had been a flood making it brown with silt. Although it was in full spate, it was not threatening, but was beautiful and sublime. The steady, drumming cascade was peaceful. The place was full of an atmosphere of serenity and worship. Marilyn and I discussed the possibility of spending a longer time there, or even living there. We went for a walk beside the sea. Great brown waves were crashing down into a sort of trough which had been dug beside the sea-wall, along the promenade. Although the mighty waves pounded upon this, they were controlled by falling into this huge moat, and were broken up and washed away. You could come quite close to the edge of the falling breakers without any danger.

The atmosphere of this dream was peaceful and refreshing. I awoke with a sense of having received a revelation, of having been in an awe-inspiring presence. Could this dream be a foil to the ominous one about the sinking vessel? There, the waters were sullen and heavy. Here, although no less powerful, they are cascading with movement, energy and control. In one dream I am being submerged. In the other, I am being elevated and renewed. I feel that these are big dreams.

Reaching into Clouds   *27 October 1983*

My peace of mind is disturbed by a sort of daydream in which I go home one day to find that Thomas is enshrouded in an inky-black cloud. This completely surrounds him. He looks like a little, sooty pillar of smoke. Everywhere he goes, this cloud goes with him. He moves about the house as if he were this little pillar of smoke. I hear his voice coming out, and when I put my hand into the cloud, I can feel his face, his body, his hair. He is there all right. I can feel his jumper, tell what he is wearing. When I withdraw my hand, there is nothing. His voice, and the noises of everything that he is doing come out of the smoke.

Now I notice that Lizzie is the same. She is a smaller pillar of smoke. When they are sitting next to each other, the two black patches merge. I can hear the clinks and the movement of the toys with which they are playing. But to really tell what they are doing, I have to stretch my hand into the blackness. I imagine myself blowing at it, trying to puff it away, but nothing will shift it.

Coming home on a later day Marilyn is also enclosed within a black cloud. I am horrified. I have to reach my hand into the cloud to see if she's had her hair done, whether she is wearing earrings. Then friends arrive. I discover to my surprise that they can see through these black clouds. The black clouds are in me. It is not the children who are under some mysterious curse but myself.

Walking home from work on a later evening, I find that the whole house is surrounded by a black cloud. I go in, through the door. There is a murky blackness inside. Nothing will dissipate it. It does not seem to make any difference whether the lights are on or not. Everything in the house is engulfed by it, but only to me, not to anyone else. Next day, the whole world has been immersed by the cloud.

This fantasy troubles me. I have been thinking to myself that I am not a blind person, but a sighted person who cannot see. In this fantasy I have to realize that the blindness is inside me. The black cloud is in my brain. It surrounds my consciousness.

Does Thomas Know I Am Blind?   *22 November 1983*

Thomas and I were playing with a little plastic turtle, about three inches in diameter. He slid it behind my glasses, covering my left eye and said, in a teasing voice, 'Now Daddy can't see with that eye. Daddy can only see with *that* eye,' pointing to the right eye. He then removed the turtle from my left eye, laughed and remarked, 'Now Daddy can see again.'

In all of our human relationships, there is a natural assumption of reciprocity. I speak and I expect you to speak. I extend my hand and I expect you to extend your hand. I smile, I expect you to return my smile. So it is with sight. I see you, I expect that you see me.

Marilyn has often remarked that I tend to play with the children in a dark room, having forgotten to turn the lights on. We are often amused by the fact that the children accept this without comment, as if it were perfectly normal. Last Monday night I took Thomas upstairs into my study intending to listen to a cassette together. We went into the room, I closed the door. The curtains were drawn and it was, in any case, pitch dark outside. I made no comment nor did Thomas. He sat down on my knee, we got out the cassettes and I put one or two on the deck in order to locate the track I wanted. Having found it, I suggested to Thomas that he should find the corresponding pictures in the book which went with the cassette. He got down, went across towards the shelf where the books are kept, then hesitated, moved towards the light switch by the door, and said, 'Thomas wants the light. Thomas can't see without the light.'

It occurred to me afterwards that the implications of this are that Thomas thinks I can see in the dark. He can't see without the lights on; I can see whether it's light or dark.

I do not suppose that he has actually formed this thought in his mind as a sentence, that I can see in the dark, but it may well be the taken-for-granted belief which is the presupposition of his behaviour with me. He is, after all, perfectly used to the idea that adults can do things which he cannot do. I, as Daddy, can lift things which are too heavy for him. It would seem only natural that I, as Daddy, can see in conditions where he cannot see. After all, it might be said that I behave exactly as if I really can see in the dark. I never ask to have the light put on, and never bother about whether it is on or not.

How, then, does Thomas construe his relationship with me? He would assume reciprocity. As he is to me, so I am to him. He would also assume my superiority. Anything he can do, I can do better.

Imogen, who is now about ten and a half years old, seems to have forgotten that so recently I was able to see. She made a reference to the fact that when I was a little boy I could see. She seemed surprised when Marilyn and I laughed and corrected her. Marilyn reminded her that I could see when I was a grown man. Only a few days ago Imogen and I were reminiscing about something we had done together which clearly involved me being able to see.

Misunderstandings   *26 November 1983*

Many misunderstandings arise from sighted people's difficulties in realizing the problems of blind mobility.

My route by foot to and from the office takes me past the University gates on the Bristol Road. These consist of a large set of double gates used by the traffic, and two smaller gates, one either side, used by pedestrians.

The other evening, I was approaching the little right-hand gate. Somebody called out, 'Hang on, mate, that gate's closed. You'll have to use this one.' Had I been sighted and had only just noticed that the gate was closed, I would simply have changed my route, cutting in a diagonal across the drive towards the open, left-hand gate. As a blind person, it would be more difficult to do this. I can only calculate the precise angle of the change of course if I know exactly how many steps I am from the right-hand gate. My most certain way of locating the left-hand gate is to continue the present course until I meet the line of closed gates. I must then work my way along them, until I come to the open left-hand gate. 'Thank you,' I called out 'I'll use the other gate then.' I kept walking in the same direction, towards the closed gate. My new acquaintance then thought I must be stupid as well as blind. He called, 'No, that is the one that's closed. You want this one.' 'Yes,' I replied in a friendly confident voice. 'Thanks for telling me that. This is my route for getting to the other gate, you know.' This was met by complete silence. I presumed that my would-be helper, totally baffled by my idiocy, was watching me with helpless concern, or had walked away, sadly shaking his head.

Here's another example. The other night a friend was driving me home. He pulled up near the house and asked me exactly where I would like to be dropped. 'All I need to know', I said, 'is whether I have to walk a little bit up the hill or a little bit down. So if you drop me ten or fifteen yards from my front gate and tell me whether to walk up or down, it'll be perfect.' 'I'll do better than that,' he replied cheerfully, 'I'll pull up exactly opposite your front gate.'

Unknown to my helpful friend, he was creating a problem. If I have to walk exactly opposite, I have no margin of error. If, in walking the several yards from the parked car across the footpath to my gate, I happen to err slightly, even by a few feet, and miss the gate, I have no immediate way of knowing whether I am a little too far to the right or the left. To find this out, I have to feel the fences and hedges. My friend in his car, seeing this, will conclude that I am fumbling about and get out of the car to come and help me, to my embarrassment.

If, however, he had dropped me some clear distance from the gate, telling me which way to walk, there would have been absolutely no problem, because I then have a margin of error. I can make contact with the line of fences or hedges at more or less any point, turn in the required direction, and know that within a few more paces I will encounter my familiar front gate. I am able to do this reasonably gracefully, with only a few swings of my cane. He would have succeeded in placing me on one of my routes.

So, in trying to be helpful, my friend had imposed upon me a route requiring an accuracy which is difficult for a blind person.

Playing the Recorder   *30 November 1983*

I dreamt that I was a member of a small orchestra. I was playing the recorder. We were about to play, perhaps to rehearse, or even to perform a Christmas song, carol or hymn composed by Simon Rattle, the conductor of the City of Birmingham Symphony Orchestra. We were gathering on the stage. Our music stands were in front of us. I was in a terrible state because I could not read the music. I was blind. I had no idea what I should play. There was a part for the solo recorder, and I was very nervous about what I would do when it came to this part. I got as far as telling somebody else in the orchestra about my problem. We were just beginning to discuss what I would do, whether I would be able to bluff my way through, when the dream ended.

The inconsistencies in this dream are very noticeable. Although I could not make anything out at all of the music itself, I did have a very distinct visual impression of the photocopied, handwritten transcript of the words, the lyrics which somebody was to sing. I could even read some of the words. The dream itself was very visual, and later in the same night I had another dream, in which I was getting Thomas ready for an outing. I was combing his hair, and had the most vivid impression of his features. I saw his face with the utmost clarity.

In spite of its inconsistencies, this musical dream marks an important step. For the first time I am in a situation where blindness is recognized to be the cause of a crisis. In the dream, I knew it was because of my blindness. It was a social situation, it was a question of competence, the fear was of a public disgrace and of letting one's colleagues down, and I had a terrible panicky feeling of helplessness. Is this a phallic dream?

Let us distinguish between the way that blindness affects the process of dreaming, and the way it affects the contents of the dream. In referring to the process, how does one dream about people for whom there is no visual image. Does one continue to dream in colour? How does one dream of places when there are no pictures to give form to those places? By the content, I mean the way in which the actual story of the dream recognizes blindness, whether in the dream I encounter the problems of blindness, or know myself as being blind or do things only a blind person would do, like placing my hand on someone's head to tell his or her height.

In the Public Library   *23 December 1983*

I dreamt that I was in a public library, possibly in Melbourne. I was blind because I was having various problems in sorting out my books. The librarian was helping me. Another blind man appeared. I could tell he was blind because he was carrying big boxes of what appeared to be books on tape. He had these on a large, wooden tray and, since both his hands were holding the tray, he was manoeuvring his way with difficulty between the desks and tables. He was bumping from one to another, on his way to his own desk. The books on his tray stood out vividly. They seemed to be in cardboard cases. Perhaps they were big, reel-to-reel tapes. He had cut the dust-jackets of the books up, and pasted them on to the spines of his tape boxes, so they looked just like the actual books. They were delightfully coloured, in blue, green, yellow and red. With envy and surprise, I noticed that he had a number of substantial reference books, including the *Shorter Oxford English Dictionary* and one or two other such volumes. I wondered whether he would let me copy his tapes, so that I could use them myself. In the meantime, I had found my way to my own desk, where I was doing some work on children's literature. I thumbed my way through a number of children's books, and then settled down to study a critical review. I worked my way into the first chapter, having some difficulty, because I was blind. I was not, however, using any optical aid, and the whole library scene around me was vividly portrayed.

The blind man with his tapes, could it have been me? And yet I, another blind reader, was observing him.

Panic in a Mineshaft   *6 January 1984*

The first experience of panic which I had in connection with blindness took place in the middle of December 1981. I was about to leave Birmingham for a fortnight's study in Cambridge. It was a bitterly cold winter's afternoon, and snow had been predicted. I decided that I had better get out of the house and on my way before the snow came. It was coming from the west, and with a bit of luck, I might get to Cambridge before it.

I left the house, but had only gone a hundred yards when I became aware of a growing feeling of doubt. I became intensely aware of the fact that I was walking through nothing. It was a very interesting, cold nothing. I worked my way along the lines of the fences, wanting to take my gloves off so I could feel them better, but knowing it would be too cold. The feeling that I was going nowhere grew stronger. I was alone, entering the night of an endless tunnel of intense cold. I knew that once I went in I would not be able to come back. I would be lost. I had a sense of impending doom. By now, I must be near the pedestrian traffic lights. Here I must cross the road. I leant for a moment on the iron railings by the footpath. Everything was so still. I struggled against the fear, but could not go on.

I turned and retraced my steps to the house, trying not to run, knowing that I could not run. Re-entering the house, I told Marilyn that I had felt a little unwell, and would lie down for a while. I set out again later in the day, this time successfully.

I used to have a feeling of panic in 1982 during months when I was having warm baths with oil, for the benefit of my skin. In the bath, I would have a sense of being enclosed, of being nothing but a body floating in space. The bath was supposed to last for twenty minutes, but it was a terrible effort of will to stay there for that long. I made myself count the seconds, then the minutes and refused to let myself reach out a hand to the talking clock until I knew that I must have been there for at least half the required time. The last five minutes were always the worst.

The third type of panic I have experienced in recent months is associated with the breathlessness of asthma. This is rare, but rather frightening. A day or two before Christmas I had been a little short of breath for an hour or so during the evening. I went upstairs about eleven o'clock at night and this gave me a slight wheeze. Reaching the bedroom, I sat on the edge of the bed. I was suddenly aware that my hands, my forehead and, indeed, my whole body were perspiring. I had an intense feeling of being enclosed. I desperately needed to get out. I must get out. I felt that I was banging my head, my whole body, against a wall of blindness. I had to break through this black curtain, this dark veil which surrounded me. Somewhere, out there, there was a world of light. I had to get out into it. At the same time, I had a sense of outrage. How could this happen to me? How could it be possible? What right had they? Who could ask me to go through this? Who had the right to deprive me of the sight of my own children at Christmas time?

I was filled with a sense of the unreality of the outside world. Only my body, sitting on the edge of the bed, was real. Out there, somewhere, there was supposed to be a house. I knew that, if I moved my body, I would feel parts of that house, bit by bit, as I moved my body along it. There would be corners, walls, wallpaper, surfaces, but until I did that, it was not there. All the people in it, the voices, the sound of the piano being played downstairs, everything floated as if coming from another world, another planet. Only I was there. I was real but this was all drifting away.

The difficulty I was having in breathing because of the asthma led to an associated sense of being attacked. I felt that I was being strangled, suffocated by the blackness. I was in a hot box, there was no light or air. This increased my compulsion to break out and to get away. I was trapped in a little place.

There was a persistent image which bothered me quite a bit during the early months and years of my blindness. This now came back with great power and oppressed me. I am in a little coal-truck in a mineshaft. This opens off the side of a hill. In I go, being trundled deeper and deeper into the hillside. Looking back, I can still see the light. I can see the opening of the shaft. There is a round window of light at the end of the tunnel. We are trundling further and further into the mountain. We are on a level surface, not going down, but going further and further in. The little round circle of daylight is getting smaller and smaller. I know that whoever is driving the train of little coal buckets will stop soon. It can't just go on and on like this. At any moment trucks will slow down, pause and reverse. The little well of light will start to enlarge. But no, this does not happen. Are we out of control? Is there nobody driving? Is nobody in a position to stop it? I must get out. I have to jump out. I must run back. This is not possible. The little trucks remorselessly carry me in, deeper and deeper.

Now I become aware of the weight of mountain overhead. It hides the light, the day, the air. I am still trundling deeper and deeper into the weight, into the solidity of it. I cannot even orientate myself by the slightest pinprick of light. I know now that between me and the world there lies this mountain of rock, or this impenetrable mass of smoky veil which is heavy and hot like the rock itself. I am trapped in an intolerable hiding place.

With steady controlled breathing, and by holding a small object in my hands, these feelings of panic pass away within a few minutes. I am left rather shaky, and not far from tears.

3

Beyond Light and Darkness

Winter 1983

Food and Sex   *7 January 1984*

Early in infancy we learn to associate our desires with the visual images of the things which satisfy them. So complete is the identification of desire with image that it becomes difficult to distinguish between 'I feel hungry' and 'I want to eat that food which I see there'. One feels hungry, of course, even when there is no food in sight, but once the food can be seen desire for the actual food takes the place of the feeling of hunger, or blends with the feeling, so that one's energies, attentions, senses of smell and taste are occupied with the anticipation of the perceived food. The internal sensation of hunger is now given an objective reference outside the body. Desire becomes specific. Indeed, the sight of the food can actually make you feel hungry, or make you realize that you are hungry.

This close association between image and desire reminds us that sight is an anticipatory sense. The anticipation of satisfied hunger replaces the sensation of hunger itself. As the need and its fulfilment come into focus upon the image of food, activity is aroused. I stretch out my hand for the food. I enter the restaurant. I buy the grapes. Naturally, sight is not the only sense to be involved in this. The smell of food is very important, indeed, perhaps even for sighted people the smell of food may be more

43

important than the sight. As always, however, sight is the foundation upon which the other senses build. The delicious smell of cooking attracts you to the kitchen and makes you feel hungry, but it is the sight of the food which actually tells you what is for dinner. The aroma, although wonderfully evocative, is often rather general. You say, 'That smells delicious. What is it?' Moreover, there are many foods the sight of which is much more stimulating than the smell. It is the sight of a rosy, shining apple which is attractive. The beautiful but subtle aroma of the apple, so noticeable when you open a whole crate or go into the loft where they are stored, may not be noticeable in the case of a single apple, especially when it is in the bowl with other kinds of fruit. Blindness dislocates this primordial union of desire and image. I am often bored by food, feel that I am losing interest in it or cannot be bothered eating. At the same time, I have the normal pangs of hunger. Even whilst feeling hungry, I remain unmotivated by the approach of food. I know it is there, because somebody tells me. Somebody says, 'Your soup has come', or 'Don't start yet; the waiter is working his way round the table with the vegetables.'

'But what is it?' I ask. 'It's veal cutlet.' Now I know. But what do I know? I have this sentence, and I believe it, but the visual cues which excite the actual desire and turn it outwards towards the object are lacking.

Something rather similar seems to happen in the case of sexual desire. There is, I think, the same connection between the general but disorientated sense of sexual hunger and the particular image of the one who can satisfy it. The image of that which satisfies is quite inseparable from the realization of the desire itself. What can we imagine of the sexual feelings of Adam before he met Eve? He knew he wanted something, but he did not know what. When he saw Eve, the restlessness of an unformed longing was turned into the passionate pursuit of a particular person.

So it is possible, I think, for a heterosexual blind man to be bored by women and yet to be conscious of sexual hunger. The trace of a perfume and the nuance of a voice are so insubstantial when compared with the full-bodied impact upon a sighted man of the appearance of an attractive woman. It must take a long time for a man who loses sight in adult life to transfer the cues of sexual arousal from the visual to the other senses. There must be many men in that position who wonder whether they will ever again be capable of genuine sexual excitement.

This dissociation of desire from image is a very curious and unsettling thing.

To Accept or not to Accept   *8 January 1984*

Recent experiences of panic make me think that, although I am reluctant to admit it, blindness is, for me, a kind of religious crisis. I do not have the calm and trustful acquiescence which is supposed to be the experience of those who lead the life of faith. This childlike acceptance and obedience is felt most deeply, so I have heard religious people say and have experienced myself in the past, during times of sharpest adversity.

If I were to accept this thing, if I were to acquiesce, then I would die. It would be as if my ability to fight back, my will to resist were broken. On the other hand, not to acquiesce, not to accept, seems futile. What I am refusing to accept is a fact.

This then is the dilemma. I am in the presence of an unacceptable reality.

I must be content with little answers. This requires the careful planning of each day, which must be broken into its compartments. Each hour must have its particular skills, its various techniques, its little routines which enable something to be accomplished successfully. Otherwise, I will have a sense of pointless desolation, a feeling of being carried helplessly deeper and deeper into it. This becomes so sharp that I am almost overwhelmed. The sense of subterranean or subconscious weight oppresses me, and I link in my mind the dream image of the huge, water-soaked hulk being dragged down into the depths with my waking reverie about the little coal-truck being driven remorselessly deeper and deeper beneath the infinite weight of the mountain. The common feature is irresistible heaviness.

One fights such a thing by minute steps. One adopts tiny techniques which help one to do tiny things step by step. I will not try to get home; that is too far. But I will get to the end of the next block. I cannot recover my grasp of the dictionaries and the encyclopaedias. Nevertheless, I will find out the meaning of this one word. To read the whole of this book, at this speed, will take an age. Very well, I will not even attempt it. But I will get to the bottom of this page even if it kills me.

In Houston I met a fine Catholic priest. I attached myself to his elbow, while we walked around the grounds of Rice University. We talked about the problem of not getting much done in a day. I told him about my own approach, to set little, immediate goals, and to feel pleased if, at the end of the day, I had read as much as three or four pages. He agreed. He told me that, at the end of every day, he looks around his office, with all of its chairs, and scattered papers, open books and unanswered correspondence, and he kneels at his desk and he prays,

'Lord, if there has been anything in this day's work which is of lasting worth, it is yours.' I feel that this is right. I am not expected to solve the problem of blindness. If I can take one step, it is yours.

I must also fight back by recognizing the circumstances in which panic is likely to occur. Let me see if I can set these out in my mind. I never have feelings of panic in my office. I always have a sense of being in an ordered environment, I know where things are, and I have something to get on with. I may sometimes feel sleepy and depressed, as if I can't be bothered, but I never panic.

I must carefully consider the implications of the Christmas set-up at home. Because of the pressure on sleeping space, I had had to give up my study, which I did gladly. But then I had nowhere to go, nowhere to get on with some little piece of work which would keep my brain ticking over. I must also have been affected by the fact that the whole house, from top to bottom, was littered with unfamiliar objects, children's toys all over the floor, suitcases and relatives to be bumped into. The unusual number of people in the house adds to the problem. I have to concentrate just that little bit harder to make sure that I have instant recognition. All this makes me feel that I am in an environment which is slipping out of control. I start to feel that it is swimming around me, that the unpredictable is confronting me at every step. It makes me realize the inflexibility of blind people, or I should say, the inflexible kind of life which is imposed upon people by blindness. Familiarity, predictability, the same objects, the same people, the same routes, the same movement of the hand in order to locate this or that: take these away, and the blind person is transported back into the infantile state where one simply does not know how to handle the world, how to enter into it and to control it, how to exist in a relationship with that world, where the hard-won balance between trust and fear threatens to be upset, and one is overwhelmed by the thought that the world to which one seeks to be related is unrelatable to, because either it is unreal or unavailable. It is inhabited by beings to whom it does belong, the sighted. The world which remains is then one's own body, the introspective consciousness. This is a world into which the sighted cannot penetrate, a place where some kind of inner control can be established. This is to go back beyond infancy into the unborn state, where one is free-floating without distinction, enclosed at the end of the tunnel, without a world and finally without a self.

The alternative to this is to establish some sort of environment, a study, a room, a route, a passage, some kind of territory. I wonder if this whole thing can be thought of in terms of territorial rights.

Blindness takes away one's territorial rights. One loses territory. The span of attention, of knowledge, retracts so that one lives in a little world. Almost all territory becomes potentially hostile. Only the area which can be touched with the body or tapped with the stick becomes a space in which one can live. The rest is unknown.

I am also haunted by the thought that it must be much more awful for those who, having lost their sight, go on to lose hearing as well.

Face to Face   *11 January 1984*

People sometimes ask me if I would like to feel their faces, but the face when felt is quite different from the face when seen. One of the most significant features of the face, the eyes themselves, cannot easily be touched. Moreover, the significance of the face-to-face position is becoming dim. It is the sight of the face which requires it to have a certain position. In the sighted world, it is a mark of courtesy and attention to turn one's face towards the person who is speaking, but in the blind world it does not matter. A blind person, after all, only knows you have been listening to him when you reply, not by whether you were looking at him while he was addressing you. The relationship, in other words, is no longer symbolized by the mutual position of the faces. Sight deals with spaces, with areas, and hence with positions.

What is the sexual significance of this? The face-to-face position is important in the lovemaking of sighted people, because it indicates the attention of the one turned fully upon the other. It represents the mutuality and the personal nature of the sexual exchange. There was a film about prehistoric people. One of the most dramatic scenes was when a couple making love abandoned the position, which the film shows as being universal, in which the male partner is behind the female, for the face-to-face position.

This is portrayed as the development of mere sexual intercourse into an act of communion between two persons. For the blind lover, however, the face-to-face position can no longer have the same significance for personal communion as it must have for the sighted partner. I do not think that a sighted person could easily accept this. It is such an infringement of this powerful convention about the relationship between personality and the body. How does blindness affect lovemaking? Must not blind lovers become more primitive? Must they not regress, as it were, to the situation described in the film as being pre-personal? On the other hand, is it not possible that the blind person, dependent so heavily upon touch, smell and taste, might develop new gentleness and sensitivity in that situation which is tactile all over?

Another aspect of this is the horror of being faceless, of forgetting one's own appearance, of having no face. The face is the mirror-image of the self.

Is this linked with the desire which I sometimes feel quite strongly to hide my face from others? I find I want to hold my chin and to cover my mouth with one hand, pressing my hand against my nose, as if I was wearing a mask. Is this a primitive desire to find some kind of equality? Since your face is not available to me, why should my face be available to you? Or does it spring from a sense that the face has been lost? Am I somehow mourning over the loss of the face? Am I trying to regain the assurance that I have got a face by feeling it with my own hands? I want to touch my very lips as I am speaking. Other people's voices come from nowhere. Does my own voice also come from nowhere?

I often want to rest my chin upon one of my pointed fingers, so as to remind myself always to point my face in the direction from which the sound or voice is coming. I need to do this even when in deep conversation with one person. Am I afraid that my head will develop that characteristic blind person's wobble?

The disappearance of the face is only the most poignant example of the dematerialization of the whole body. People become mere sounds. This leads to something else. Just because there is nothing to mediate between the intangible sounds of voices and the immediate contact of bodies, body-contact becomes all the more startling. A handshake or an embrace becomes a shock, because the body comes out of nowhere into sudden reality.

This comes home vividly in the experience of drinking very cold water from a tap. The impact is so immediate. All of a sudden, it is there – water! It slaps against the lips, swamps the face, floods the mouth and the stomach with its sharp presence, with no warning or preparation. It just comes smack. So is the transition from speech to body contact in the human relations of the blind person. So for blind people, other people have become both more abstract and more concrete, with an abrupt transition from one to the other. This takes us back to the problem of the sexual relationships of blind people. Perhaps blind lovers are both more abstract and more concrete, perhaps they are both more primitive and more sophisticated, in different ways. Perhaps this is what they mean when they say that true love is blind.

Who Smiled? 13 January 1984

The philosopher Paul Ricoeur has interesting things to say in his various books about the difference between speaking and writing. In the situation of speech, you are face to face. When you read something, you are no longer face to face with the author, who may have died centuries ago, or be living in a far-off land. When you are speaking face to face with someone, there is not often a problem of interpretation, because the situation itself usually makes it clear. If in doubt, you can ask the speaker what was meant.

Written materials are much less clear. The situation which gave rise to the writing may be long forgotten, or the intentions of the writer may not be understood. This is why interpretation becomes necessary, to bridge the gulf between the reader and the text. When you are face to face with the speaker, the task of interpretation is much simpler. You do not need to ask who smiled; the smiler is before you. You do not need to ask if someone is raising a hand. Intentions, speech, bodily movement and meaning are simultaneously present.

For blind people, however, there is a distance between speech and meaning, a bit like the distance between the printed text and its meaning. Just as one must try to interpret people's printed words, so blind people often find a need to interpret spoken words.

'Would you like this?' someone asks. How can a blind person interpret such a remark? For the sighted listener, the meaning is provided by the situation as it is seen. The intention of the speaker is clear because the words and the posture, what is being held out are unified. The blind person, however, does not know whether the speaker is pointing at something rather than holding out something.

Contrary to Paul Ricoeur's comment, the blind person often has to ask 'Who said that?' and such questions as 'Who smiled? Who raised their hands?' would hardly ever arise, because the blind person would not know that these actions had taken place at all. Being blind is thus a situation which has to both interpret and be interpreted.

Loss 2 February 1984

Last night I had a nightmare so vivid that it woke me up. I dreamt that Elizabeth, who will be two on 23 February, was not in her cot. Instead it was full of flowers, beautiful flowers. They were in a formal arrangement, like wreaths on a grave-stone. I went to Marilyn and said, 'Where's Lizzie?'

Marilyn said, 'She's dead.'

I was appalled, and broke down in tears, crying out, 'What happened? I didn't know. Tell me!'

Marilyn was very calm. She said, 'It's no good making a fuss. She's buried.'

I was furious. I grabbed her by the shoulders, and shook her fiercely, shouting out, 'What do you mean? How dare you! Is she not only dead but buried, and I not even told?'

Marilyn pointed out of the window. There was a grassy plot, like a cathedral close or a cloister. Over this a slow procession was moving on foot. 'There they go,' Marilyn said. 'There's the funeral procession.'

So I woke up.

This dream was very visual. The colours were brilliant, people's clothes, the green of the grass and the bright colours of the flowers. There was no trace of blindness. Who is running my children's lives? How would I even know? Did the dreamer get the names wrong? Was it, perhaps, not Lizzie and Marilyn but other people whom I have also lost? Was it Imogen who was dead, lost first through divorce and distance and lost again through the isolating effect of blindness? The many faces of loss are terrifying.

'My Husband Is Blind'   4 February 1984

Today the family went to Coventry Cathedral. Marilyn and Thomas went together to buy tickets for the special exhibition, while I remained in the coffee bar. Marilyn asked if there was a concession for disabled people, adding, 'My husband is blind.' As soon as she had got the tickets, Thomas said to her, 'Why is your husband blind?' Marilyn, in telling this to me later, said that she was most taken aback at this question, and could not help wondering if she should have said what she did say in his hearing. She replied, however, 'Because Daddy can't see.'

He then asked, 'Is Daddy your husband?'

'Yes.'

'Why can't he see?'

'Because there's something wrong with his eyes.'

Marilyn told me that Thomas did not pursue this any further, but later, as we were walking around the cathedral itself, he came over to me. This was the first time I had been alone with him, although Marilyn had already told me what had happened. 'Daddy,' he asked me, 'are you blind?' I took him in my arms, and said, 'Who's been telling you that?'

This was a foolish and evasive answer and I do not quite know why

I said it. In some obscure way that I cannot fully understand I felt ashamed. I was fearful that some change in my relationship with him might take place. Anyway, he now knows I am blind. Does he, however, know what blindness is? What conclusions will he be able to draw from his knowledge that I am blind?

'When I Close My Eyes You Can't See Me'   *9 February 1984*

Marilyn told me that yesterday whilst Thomas was playing with Lizzie he closed his eyelids very tightly, saying to her, 'When I close my eyes you can't see me.' He kept his eyes closed for some seconds, while Lizzie stared at him, wide-eyed with wonder. Finally he opened his eyes and said triumphantly, 'There!' This is a vivid example of the assumption of reciprocity. One assumes that the other is like oneself. Not to see is the same as not to be seen. The active and the passive forms of speech are collated. Not to see is thus to be unobserved. A blind person is invisible. A person who closes his own eyes is also invisible. No one can see him. If one does not use sight, one is not available for sight. The argument from reciprocity runs like this: I can see Daddy; Daddy is therefore not invisible; therefore Daddy can see.

It would be all too easy to dismiss this as a piece of infantile reasoning. We should remember the so-called 'illusion of privacy', a feature of the behaviour of many blind adults. It refers to the difficulty of remembering all the time, when you are blind, that you can be seen. It is so hard always to bear in mind the astonishing range of this faculty which other people are said to have. The blind person has to remind himself all the time, when tempted to scratch his bum, that he is visible.

This is not the case when hearing is lost. I have never heard of a child who put his fingers in his ears and shouted 'You can't hear me.' One of the reasons for this, I think, is that the organ of hearing and that of speech are located separately on the head or the face. The organ by means of which one hears (the ears) and the organs by means of which one makes oneself heard (the larynx and the mouth) are not identical. The organ with which one sees and the organ with which one is seen are, however, identical. Sight is reciprocal but hearing is sequential.

The eye is thus related both actively and passively to other eyes, which is not the case with the ear, which is an organ of receptivity only.

Touch is reciprocal under normal conditions. If I can feel you, you can normally feel me feeling you. If I cannot feel you, it is probable that you cannot feel me. The difference between touch and sight is that the reciprocity of sight can be turned off so easily. There are ways of turning off the reciprocity of mutual touch. I could feel you while you were asleep, or I could hold a lock of your hair without you becoming aware of it. You might have had a dab of anaesthetic and your skin might be dulled. In the case of sight, however, you only have to close your eyes. The closing of the eyes is a normal, indeed, a moment by moment action, whereas the shutting off of the sense of touch is not so simple.

The implications of this reciprocity of sight for the relationships between the blind and the sighted are extensive. Because I cannot see, I cannot be seen. I can be ignored, treated as if I did not exist, spoken about in the third person. 'Will you look after him?' 'Will you put him by the lift?' 'Where would you like to sit him?' 'Will you walk him back to his office?' When in a hurry, one can rush past a blind friend without the inconvenience of having to greet him. He does not see you, therefore he does not know. Therefore you can pretend that you cannot see him either.

The other day, with my colleague Michael Grimmitt, I was interviewing a student. Michael told me afterwards that she did not look at me once during the entire interview. All of her questions, her smiles, her whole body were pointed towards Michael. Even when I was directly questioning her, she barely inclined her head in my direction.

Was it that she could not bear to look at me? Did she think that Michael would think she was stupid if she smiled at me and looked at me because she would know that Michael would know that I could not know if she smiled at me or not? Whatever the reason, the effect was that she was unable to see me, because I was unable to see her.

This feeling of having become invisible must be related to the loss of the body image. Just as one has lost the faces of others, so it would not matter if one's own face were to be lost. On cold, wintry mornings, I suffer from a strange, almost inhuman feeling, that I could go around not merely with the lower part of my face muffled against the wind, but with my entire head shrouded. It would make no difference if my whole face disappeared. Being invisible to others, I become invisible to myself. This means that I lack self-knowledge, I become unconscious. This is what the archetype of blindness indicates, the loss of consciousness, the descent into sleep, the sense of nothingness, of becoming nothing. To be seen is to exist.

This gives insight into the longing of the beloved sighted to be seen by the beloved blind. It is the longing to exist in the lover's sight, the desire to be perceived by him. This is surely what lies behind the thought which my elder daughter, aged ten and a half, expressed the other day,

'Oh Daddy, I wish you could *see* me.' This is not merely the desire to be seen performing some feat, such as a younger child might feel, it is the desire to have been in the presence of someone who did, as a parent, confer being, but now is blind.

Rapunzel   *11 February 1984*

The other day Thomas and I were listening to the story of Rapunzel on cassette. When we came to the part where the young prince falls from the tower, scratches his eyes on the thorns and becomes blind, Thomas interrupted, in some agitation, turning to me and crying out, 'Why was he blind?'

'Because the thorns hurt his eyes,' I replied.

'Why did the thorns hurt his eyes?'

'It was when he fell out of the tower. He fell on to the thorn bushes.'

There was a pause while he digested this. I decided to take the initiative. 'What's blindness, Thomas?'

After a short pause, he replied thoughtfully, 'I don't know.'

There was again a short pause. The illustration in the book apparently showed the young prince wandering through the forest with a white cane or a stick of some kind, because Thomas next asked, 'Is the prince blind?'

'Yes,' I replied.

Thomas added, 'He's carrying a stick.'

'Is it a white stick?' I asked him.

'No.'

'Why is he carrying a stick?' I inquired.

Again there was a pause, and he said, 'I don't know.'

Thomas does not know what the word 'blind' means, although he realizes that it is something to do with one's eyes. He knows that it is not natural, and is, indeed, the result of some misfortune, and he knows that blindness is associated with the carrying of a stick, although it is not clear quite what the association is. He made no reference to my own blindness, nor to the conversation we had last week which so startled him, when he heard Marilyn say that her husband was blind. Is it possible that my foolish refusal to answer his question directly, about whether I was indeed blind, has now confused him? Perhaps he now is not quite sure whether I am blind or not. He does, however, realize that the word 'blind' is a significant word for us all.

Blindness as an Archetype   *23 February 1984*

Blindness is the archetype of the loss of consciousness. Light suggests intelligence and knowledge; darkness suggests chaos and ignorance. In the blind person, one confronts the symbol of the loss of the ordered, intelligent life. Our conscious lives emerge slowly and painfully out of our unconscious, pre-natal selves, and the loss of conscious life remains one of our deepest anxieties.

This may help us to understand why sighted people are usually so amazed to find that blind people can do anything at all. They expect that, with the loss of consciousness, blind people would be engulfed by a sense of lostness, of wandering helplessly, of confusion and indistinction.

The sighted person who goes blind confronts in his or her own person the actual presence of the archetype which had been dimly feared. The archetype will now be activated, not by being confronted in a stranger, but by being a fact of one's own daily experience. Perhaps this helps us to understand better the panic which a recently blinded person can so easily feel. In my own case, the feeling of being bricked up inside comes into conflict with the fear that there is no reality outside, and that one is trapped, on the borderlands between the real and the unreal, where all is confusion and darkness. Perhaps part of the panic is the desire to get outside in order to reassure oneself that there is something there.

Fighting Depression   *24 February 1984*

Occasionally I feel depressed, and this is worst when I am frustrated in playing with the children. I feel as if I have become nothing, unable to act as a father, impotent, unable to survey, to admire, or to exercise jurisdiction or discrimination. I have a strange feeling of being dead.

My response is to go even further inwards, into a deeper deadness. I sink into quietness and passivity. I might sit in a chair alone, without moving, reducing my breathing to the barest minimum, simmering down until I am aware of less and less. I try to think of nothing, and often drift in and out of sleep. I might cover myself with a blanket, cutting out any faint sounds, and by emptying myself completely, I become the cipher that my blindness tells me I am. In this state, I can continue for hours.

This technique for fighting depression is effective up to a point. It does provide a certain refuge, a kind of solace, a place to go to. I certainly find that, if the joyful games of the children throw me into one of these depressed states, and if I am unable to go into my nothingness refuge, possibly because I am responsible for the children and have to remain alert, or because of some social obligation to visitors or friends, then I seem to go to pieces. I build up inner tension. There is a tightness in my forehead, a feeling that I will not be able to go on much longer. The image of the quiet little bed in the corner of my study keeps flooding into my mind and I feel that the demands of the outside world which prevent me from retiring are rapidly becoming less and less acceptable. Each voice comes, as it were, from an increasingly remote distance, and is heard with increasing reluctance. The sounds of the outside world now strike me with a certain pain, as if they are preventing me from obtaining relief, and I will, at this stage, find it impossible to remain awake.

I must find another way of tackling this problem. I need to understand it more. Perhaps my imagination has come under the power of the symbolic associations of blindness. Perhaps my actual blindness has activated the archetype of blindness within me.

This could be why, in these states of depression I feel as if I am on the borders of conscious life, not just in the literal sense that I am slipping in and out of sleep, but in a deeper and more alarming sense. I feel as if I want to stop thinking, stop experiencing. The lack of a body image makes this worse: the fact that one can't glance down and see the reassuring continuity of one's own consciousness in the outlines of one's own body, moving a distant foot which, so to speak, waves back, saying, 'Yes, I hear you. I am here.' There is no extension of awareness into space. So I am nothing but a pure consciousness, and if so, I could be anywhere. I am becoming ubiquitous; it no longer matters where I am. I am dissolving. I am no longer concentrated in a particular location, which would be symbolized by the integrity of the body.

The archetype of blindness represents the power to obliterate the distinction between that which is known and that which is not known, that which is here and that which is not here, the inside and the outside, the specific and the general. It represents dissolution, the borderland between being and not-being.

The techniques which I have described for fighting panic and depression are only partly successful. In the case of the withdrawing technique, it is too similar to the object of its fear. This is why it cannot be an effective response, urgent and perhaps inevitable though it may be in the short term. As for blindness being an archetype, what do I do about it? I need to find an antidote. Could there be an opposing archetype? Could this be the idea of light? Light is certainly one of the perennial symbols.

Light gives detail, drives away uncertainty, allows discrimination, dissolves ambiguity, and gives a particular place and context.

One of the most beautiful biblical passages which expresses the power of the archetype of light is found in Numbers 6.24–6, the Aaronic Blessing: 'The Lord bless you and keep you, the Lord make his face to shine upon you and be gracious unto you, the Lord lift up the light of his countenance upon you and give you peace.' This passage expresses the clarity, the radiance and the sense of identity which is conferred by being in the presence of the lighted face of God.

Another passage which expresses the archetype of light is found in 1 John 1.5: 'God is light, and in him there is no darkness at all.'

This is of limited use to me. God may be in light but I am in darkness. This alternative archetype only oppresses me by the brightness of its contrast. By obliterating the darkness, it obliterates me. The archetype of light cancels the archetype of darkness but does not transcend it. It cannot transcend the darkness/light distinction because it is one side of it. I need to find an alternative archetype of a higher order.

Beyond Light and Darkness   26 February 1984

Thomas had asked me if he could have the light on in the room where we were playing. It had not occurred to me that it had become dark. He had explained, 'Thomas needs the light. Daddy doesn't need the light.'

I thought of the passage in Psalm 139.12: 'Darkness and light are both alike to thee.' There is a strange sense in which I have become like God. I may have discovered not so much the opposing archetype as the alternative one, the one which transcends and unifies at a higher level.

Darkness is as Light with Thee   27 February 1984

'O Lord, thou hast searched me and known me' (Ps. 139.1). This is a meditation about knowledge. God knows the posture of my body without having to touch me. 'Thou knowest when I sit down and when I rise up' (v. 2). God possesses that strange power of knowing at a distance. I am often surprised that my sighted friends know something when it is still so far off. The blind have to remember that it is just as if the sighted were touching their faces all the time. Sighted people gain knowledge of what blind people are thinking just through watching their faces. 'Thou discernest my thoughts from afar' (v. 2). Sighted people often call out, telling me that there is a car parked on the footpath.

Friends often tell me that they saw me (from their cars) crossing the road. They honked me, but there was no way I could recognize them before the traffic moved on. I was surprised the other day to find out how far down the road I was when my children, knowing I was coming, had time to prepare something for me. 'Thou searchest out my path and my lying down, and art acquainted with all my ways' (v. 3).

In some ways, God's knowledge of the world is rather like the knowledge which the sighted have of the blind, but it also goes further. 'Open your eyes!' one of my sighted friends said to her husband. 'I can't tell what you're thinking when you sit there with your eyes closed.' The eyes of the blind are inscrutable. It is true that the sighted can catch the transient emotions upon the face of the blind, but all too often I find that my friends think I am asleep, when in fact I am paying very close attention to them. I must speak if they are to know my inner thoughts. Speech becomes all important to the blind. God, however, does not depend upon my speech to know me, even though I am blind. 'Even before a word is on my tongue, lo, O Lord thou knowest it altogether' (v. 4). It is at this point that we realize that we are entering into the presence of something which transcends the distinction between blindness and sight, darkness and light.

The psalm continues with all the emotions which the blind person would have. As a sighted person, you are acknowledged by your friends with a smile, a nod, a wink or even the most fleeting exchange of glances. To be acknowledged by my friends, I must soon be spoken to or touched. I find that I have developed a little habit, which I feel sure is due to my blindness, of shaking hands with people by using both of my hands. I somehow feel the need to extend an acknowledgement of their presence which will make up for my inability to receive their smiles. When I am speaking at a meeting, it is important to go around as many people as I can beforehand, shaking hands and literally making contact. 'Thou dost beset me behind and before and layest thy hand upon me' (v. 5).

I drop a teaspoon on to the floor. I lower my twelve-month-old baby, holding her by the waist. I wait a moment, moving her up and down a little like a vacuum cleaner. I lift her up again. The teaspoon is in her hand. I am full of wonder. She picked it up, so smoothly, so easily, with no need to scrape the carpet with her hand. She went straight for it. How did she know? This child has some strange sense which I can but remember. God's knowledge fills me with even greater wonder. 'Such knowledge is too wonderful for me! It is high, I cannot attain it' (v. 6). What does 'high' mean to a blind person? How high are the buildings?

How high are the clouds? I only know that things are up there; they are beyond my reach.

The knowledge which God has is inescapable. It surrounds me; it fills me. It makes every place alike, for all places are known to God. 'Whither shall I go from thy spirit? Or whither shall I flee from thy presence?' (v. 7). There are no degrees of the divine presence because there are no degrees of divine knowledge. 'If I ascend to heaven, thou art there. If I make my bed in Sheol thou art there' (v. 8). God is Lord of all worlds. The world of heaven, of light is God's. The world of Sheol, of darkness and of the depths is also God's. It makes no difference to God where I am, or in what world I find myself. God is not enclosed within the world of heavenly light nor is God defeated by the world of impenetrable night.

Now I imagine I am flying. I imagine I am free, once again, to go where I will, and that the morning and the ocean will once again be accessible to me. 'If I take the wings of the morning and dwell in the uttermost parts of the sea . . .' (v. 9). I may, perhaps, live beneath the sea, in that world of the unconscious depths. Even there, the One who is the Lord of all worlds will make himself known to me in the manner which suits my condition. He will not show himself to me: he will not appear to me. He will not offer me a vision or be transformed in glory. He will remember my blindness. '. . . even there thy hand shall lead me and thy right hand shall hold me' (v. 10).

I feel certain that the author of this psalm was blind. Nobody else could have described so powerfully the religious experience of the blind person, or could have interpreted so perfectly the presence of a blind person before God.

We now come to the climax of the psalm. 'If I say, "Let only darkness cover me and light about me be night, even the darkness is not dark to thee. The night is bright as the day, for darkness is as light with thee" ' (vv. 11f). Sometimes I feel that I am being buried in blindness. I am being carried deeper and deeper in. The weight presses me down. Such knowledge as I have is disappearing, is so limited, so fragile, my hold upon it is so feeble. Should I then wish this? Should I accept it with some kind of spirit of sacrifice? Should I plunge myself in the inevitable, so that even my remaining knowledge will sink into ignorance?

Just as blindness has the effect of obliterating the distinctions, so the divine omniscience transcends them. Because I am never in the light, it is equally true that I am never in the darkness. I have no fear of the darkness because I know nothing else. Nobody can turn the lights out on me. So it is with God. Indifferent alike to both light and darkness

God does not need the light in order to know and the darkness cannot prevent him from knowing. In that sense, it is true that if darkness is as light, then light is as darkness. The older translation of the Authorized Version brings out the point more vividly: 'Darkness and light are both alike to thee.' This is not the image of a beam of light penetrating the darkness and banishing it. God does not overwhelm the darkness by his light; God represents that pure knowledge to which both light and darkness in their different ways point.

I come back to the one thing I know. There is my body, sitting here on the edge of the bed, trembling and sweating. There is the tension in my stomach, the pounding in my temples. I hear my breathing, I feel my heart pounding. I do not know what is out there; I know what is in here. '. . . for thou didst form my inward parts. Thou didst knit me together in my mother's womb . . . thou knowest me right well . . . my frame was not hidden from thee. When I was being made in secret intricately wrought in the depths of the earth thy eyes beheld my unformed substance. In thy book were written every one of them, the days that were formed for me when as yet there was none of them' (vv. 13ff).

The psalm remains remarkably faithful to the experience of blindness. Is it not strange that my knowledge of what is going on six inches inside me should be more accurate than my knowledge of what is going on six inches away from me? Whether inside or outside, however, all is alike to the divine knower.

The physical closeness of two people making love is a problem to the pornographic film-maker, for at the point of most intimate touching where sight becomes irrelevant, the pornographer must introduce distance in order to retain visual excitement. It is amusing for a blind man to think that there is still one thing he can do, and people often remark that you don't need speech and you don't need sight to do it. No matter how exciting and profound may be the mutual knowledge which lovers exchange, none can ever be said to know or experience the moment when the sperm joins the ovum and a new life is born. I was made in secret and I am still being made in the secrets of blindness, but all secrets are open to God. I no longer know the passage of my days by means of the alternation of day and night, light and darkness, and in this sense also, my knowledge of my days is rather like God's. The important thing about waking up is not the morning but the presence. I am restored by wakefulness to the presence of the ones I love. 'When I awake I am still with thee' (v. 18), so although I experience the paradoxes of rediscovering sight in the unconscious life of dreams and of losing my sight once again every time I wake up, the paradoxes are transcended in communion with the One who knows me, whether I wake or sleep, for I am still with him.

Not Acceptance but Praise   28 February 1984

'Wonderful are thy works . . . how precious to me are thy thoughts, O God! How vast is the sum of them! If I were to count them, they are more than the sand . . .' (Ps. 139.14ff).

As a blind person, sitting on the beach, I have poured a fistful of sand upon the palm of my other hand, allowing it to trickle through my fingers. I have rubbed the sand between my finger and thumb, wondering at the various textures. Some of the grains are coarse and sharp, filing the skin in such a way that every little speck stands out. Some are so smooth and silky that it is almost impossible to tell the grains, the sand disappearing like water. If I stretch my hand out a little further, I can still grasp sand, and so on, further and further. I know that with sight I could tell the sweep of this beach for miles around the bay. This beach is but one of thousands of such beaches, and there are probably thousands of people like me just now, doing what I am doing, running the grains between their fingers and wondering. So are the divine thoughts. My body holds them, one by one, while I feel myself held like a grain upon the hand of God. What matters is not that I am blind, but that I am known and that I am led by the hand, and that my life, whether sighted or blind, is full of praise.

Above and Below the Sea   2 March 1984

Last night I had the most powerful, frightening and impressive dream. I was on board a huge ship. There were no women on board, it was all men. It appeared to be some kind of naval expedition. Giant waves kept crashing right over the ship. The first of these we saw coming. Everyone ran for shelter. We had time to scuttle inside the bulkheads, to run along to the end, and to clamber up the metal stairways. Up and up we climbed to the very top recesses. Then the wave broke. It came crashing across the deck, into the cabins and holds, swamping the whole of the interior section where we were, and splashing right up, but not quite touching us. We were all grouped on the very top part of this spacious hall, or stateroom in the ship. This was the first of many such waves. One, in particular, I saw coming. It was a mountainous, threatening wall of dark, green water. They crashed again and again over the ship. The whole place was awash. We ourselves had just managed to escape, although others were being swept away. Now the vessel became a submarine. We went down, under the water. We were on some kind of mission. Three men seemed to be in charge. They were the captain and his helpers, the officers. They were swimming around, beautiful, strong, powerful men. Now I had an external view of this submarine. Still it was descending, very modern, like a space craft. It was covered with bulbs, all sorts of equipment and lamps. It was not particularly large, but was coming down and down, very gently. Now it was resting on the deck of another ship, far beneath the water, where there seemed to be some mission to accomplish. Then we were back inside the large vessel. There seemed to be some kind of disaster, a punishment amongst the crew. There was my colleague, Michael, being wrapped up inside a blanket or a shroud and hung on a rope out of the cabin window. This was to serve as a punishment, or some kind of signal. As he was lowered out of the window, I heard the bell sounding. I was full of distress, and I saw others of my colleagues being punished in the same way. I did not know what for. I was full of fear that somehow or other my colleagues and I had let down the expedition, disgraced the party. We were being punished in this dreadful and incomprehensible manner by these majestic men who were our captains. It was a very vivid, compelling and exciting dream.

Above and below blindness . . . is there to be a meeting with something down there? What loss! What failure! How incomprehensible it all is and how irresistible!

Am I Asleep?   *4 March 1984*

If I pause in my work, lean back in my chair, and listen to the sounds of the traffic from the street outside, I sometimes have a sort of hallucination. I see things. A visual impression will flash before my mind. Often, this is something quite trivial.

I saw a little scene in which I was standing in the back garden of a house. I was looking beyond the red brick wall of a building, possibly a garage, to the six-foot wooden fence at the back of the property. Beyond this, there was a path or an alley along which people were moving to and fro, both on foot and on bicycles. A plank was missing from the fence, and through the six-inch gap I caught glimpses of raincoats and wheels. The whole scene was intensely vivid, full of perspective, movement and colour. The outlines were crisp and clean, every detail was in place. Then it faded, and I returned to the sounds of the traffic and the feel of my machines and the thoughts about what I had been reading.

Now the question. Had I been asleep or not? Only in dreams do I have such visual experiences. I can, of course, remember what things look like, but I only forget that I am remembering, and have the actual visual experience, when I am asleep. So my dreams correspond to my earlier active, sighted life. There is a sort of in-between state, when I am conjuring up mental images, perhaps related to what someone is telling me.

If a friend is driving me through town, and happens to remark, 'We are passing through an older part of the city now, there are lots of scruffy little shops and launderettes,' then immediately before my mind comes a picture of what I imagine these streets would look like. When this happens, however, I know perfectly well that I am doing it. I am conscious of toying with various images of what the street might look like, flashing various slides on the screen, as it were, to see which might fit the description best. Similarly, if I gaze out of my office window and try to reconstruct the scene as I remember it, putting in clumps of trees here, following the noise of the traffic and picturing the streets running this way and that, trying to remember whether it was possible to see as far as such and such a building, I am conscious of the effort. Moreover, the result is patchy. Here the picture is rather incomplete, because I remember the school and the playing fields, but over here, it is more vague. What was over there? Am I confusing what can be seen from this window with the view from another window, further along or on a higher floor?

In the dreamlike hallucination, there are no gaps. Every part of the picture is completely filled in, as it is with real sight. There is no uncertainty, no speculation, no toying with alternatives and no sense of effort. I am there, as viewing that scene, which is presented to me with all the unmistakable vigour of a real world pressing in. I must conclude then, that in the little image of the back yard and the scene through the fence, I had actually been asleep and dreaming.

This disturbs me. It is as if that part of my brain which is stored with visual memories is longing to be activated, crying out to be called upon and made use of. The conscious life permits little possibility of this, so the moment there is a lapse of consciousness, the visual memories come crowding in with all the realism and compulsiveness of dreams. This, perhaps, is why in these little cameos there is seldom any plot, seldom any emotion. The overpowering feature is the visual image itself. Dreams, of course, are always based on memories, but it seems to me that blindness represents a sort of half-way state between consciousness and unconsciousness, on the borderland between dream and memory, where the distinctions between sleep and wakefulness can easily become blurred.

A Visit from a Faith Healer   *5 March 1984*

On a number of occasions in one of the Birmingham city centre churches Marilyn and I had met a man whom I will call Mr Cresswell. A few Sundays ago Mr Cresswell approached me after the morning service, shook me warmly by the hand, and told me that God had told him that it was his intention to heal me of my blindness. Mr Cresswell would have to wait for the signal from the Lord that the time had come but as soon as the Lord did give him the word he would be along to see me. I congratulated him on having received this message, adding that, as soon as the Lord gave him the word he was to lose no time but to come out and see me straight away.

He called at the house a couple of times during the following weeks but I was out. He then rang and an appointment was made for five o'clock on Friday 2 March. When I arrived home from the office, Mr Cresswell was already there talking with Marilyn. Thomas and Lizzie were frisking around rather noisily and when it became clear that we were about to start, Marilyn offered to leave the room and take the children with her. Mr Cresswell was, however, very anxious that she should remain, and so we all stayed.

Mr Cresswell began by telling me that I had had a fall when I was young. He did not deny that what the doctors said about detached retina might well be true, according to their lights, but the other way of looking at it was that I had had a fall and this had caused me to lose my sight. I expressed interest in this in a fairly non-committal way and we passed on to various other subjects. Mr Cresswell told me a little bit about his work, his calling to be a healer, and the extent of his ministry. He had special knowledge. We, for example, had a sick woman teacher friend. Marilyn and I discussed this briefly. We do have dozens of women teacher friends but, to the best of our knowledge, none of them was sick at that time. Mr Cresswell did not pursue that line of inquiry, but told us that we were missing someone very badly. We were, he told us, missing our home. He asked which home we were missing. We told him that this was our home and we were not missing any other place. 'Aren't you homesick for your parents' place?' We repeated that this was our home, we loved each other very much, we were happy together and although we loved our parents we did not miss their home. Mr Cresswell then introduced the idea that our true home was heaven, and this was the place that we should be missing.

These little attempts at clairvoyance having been somewhat inconclusive, our visitor began another explanation about my lack of sight. He told me that I had ceased to read the Bible. I assured him that I had not ceased to read the Bible and he countered this by insisting that I was not reading it as much as I used to. I informed him that I was only reading the Bible for about half an hour a day, and in braille, whereas in the past I had occasionally read the Bible more each day, and at other times less. Mr Cresswell seemed to think this a clear admission of guilt, commenting that the moment we stop reading the Bible these things come upon us. I pointed out that there are many sighted people who had stopped or who had never read the Bible. They did not lose their sight, so the thing he was describing could hardly be a general rule. Mr Cresswell pointed out that people are different, and then again maybe it was not me but my parents or grandparents because God visits their sins unto the third and fourth generation. Mr Cresswell took a vigorously punitive view of illness and disability.

These preliminaries being concluded, Mr Cresswell called for a Bible. Marilyn offered him a New English Bible, but he was not satisfied with it. We passed him an Authorized Version, which was acceptable. He sat there for some time apparently meditating on what he should read. He gave the impression that he was waiting to receive instructions because he muttered softly, 'Genesis? Yes? No, not Genesis. All right. Acts? Yes, we'll have the first chapter of Acts.'

Since I was unable to read the printed version, Marilyn was asked to read. In order to impress upon him that I had not stopped reading the Bible, I broke into the reading about half-way through the chapter and quoted from memory the following six or eight verses. Mr Cresswell was delighted with this, and Marilyn then completed the chapter. Our visitor called for a cup of cold water, stood up, asked me to remove my glasses, placed one of his hands over my forehead and eyes, sprinkled my head with the water, and prayed, first a general, healing prayer, then the Lord's Prayer, followed by the Twenty-third Psalm. He then anointed my eyes with the water, above and below each lid, and asked me to roll up my right sleeve. He was taken aback to discover that my arm was bandaged. He asked me what that was in a tone of surprise and some indignation. I explained that I had been having a little eczema and he told me to remove the bandage, and that I would never, never wear it again. I was not sure if this was an instruction or a prediction, but certainly Mr Cresswell seemed slightly upset by the bandage, possibly because I had not informed him about the full extent of my bodily state, or perhaps because his special knowledge had not revealed it to him. Be that as it may, I was then grasped by the upper arm, and Mr Cresswell made firm, stroking movements right down the arm to the tip of the fingers, stroking each finger or pulling each finger one by one to the very tip. This was repeated on my left arm and then over my head, although I cannot quite remember if the movements on the head were up or down. The evil influences having been removed from me in this way, I was then told to take cod liver oil mixed with an equal quantity of honey. Nothing was said about whether the dosage should be repeated, or how often, and I did not inquire.

This entire ritual was repeated again on Marilyn who was then commanded to drink a little bit of the remaining water and in a forceful voice I was commanded to finish it off. That was the end of the matter, and Marilyn left the room to put the two babies in the bath. Mr Cresswell remained for a few moments, and we had a very friendly and lively conversation about his work and the Lord's work. I thanked him for coming and thanked him for his prayers and readings. He told me that the Lord had seen fit to afflict me with this pain but that probably he would now see fit to remove it. He was cautious, and emphasized the probability only. So, with renewed greetings and warm embraces, together with a promise to return to offer further treatment if the Lord so instructed him, Mr Cresswell took his leave.

Raspberry Cordial   *10 March 1984*

In a situation of sharp alienation, or when I feel overcome by a sense of my own non-existence, I am visited by a sudden brilliant memory which seems to come from early childhood. The first sign of this is a vivid sensation, usually of taste, smell or touch.

I was returning in the car with the family from a meal in a restaurant. During the meal I had been troubled by a powerful feeling of unreality, and in the car on the way home I was suddenly gripped by thirst. I realized that what I was longing for, no, what I was actually tasting, was the delightful, strong, sweet flavour of a raspberry cordial which used to be given to us on Sunday School treats when I was a child. As the realization of the taste filled me, visual images began to appear. I saw the white paper cup with the deep, crimson circle of the cordial within it, before it was filled to the brim with water from the jug. Then I saw the other cups standing in rows on the wooden trestle table, with the paper tablecloth. And then the whole scene burst upon me.

I am back in a small town in the state of Victoria. We children, barefooted, have been running our races over the parched ground between the parked cars and the horses and buggies and now we come, excited and panting, to be filled up with cups of this delicious drink, to be followed by masses of sandwiches and sausage rolls.

What is surprising about this experience is how it started. It did not, like most memories of childhood, emerge in a discussion about childhood with some other adult, especially a brother or sister. It did not emerge anecdotally at all. First came the sensation. Only gradually was the sensation located, first as being raspberry cordial, then as being in a paper cup, then as being on a trestle table, until finally the whole scene unfolded and I recognized that I was thinking of something, experiencing something, which I had not thought of for forty of fifty years. But why?

Is it possible that in a state of shock one tends to go back into childhood? Is it possible that in withdrawing from the painful, present world, one retreats to a very much older and more secure layer of one's personhood? Is it possible that in retreating from the tumult of the waves, my consciousness is going deeper and deeper, and all sorts of strange and half-forgotten fish never seen at the surface levels are now coming into view?

I have another theory. Sight and hearing may be thought of as the intellectual senses. They give knowledge, without actually producing a corresponding sensation which is felt by the body. When these cognitive senses are lost, one is forced back within the body. Bodily sensations, which in normal life occupy only the very margin of awareness, take on a new interest and importance. Often, there is nothing else of which to be aware, except what is happening within one's own body. An itch, a pain, a warmth, this is all there is to think about. Moreover, there is a natural connection between this situation and that of young children. They live very immediately in their bodies. The newborn baby sees and hears, but what occupies its attention is what it feels immediately within its body, especially the stomach and the lips, made more vivid by the inability to distinguish inside from outside.

Perhaps when an adult becomes blind, there is an inner return to the body, and a discovery of all sorts of traces of early bodily experience. The spontaneous, vivid appearance of these memories gives them rather a fascinating dreamlike quality. They come unsummoned. One becomes aware of an inner population seeking expression.

These experiences have taught me something about how to remember childhood. Many adults try to inspect a collection of pictures in the memory, hoping that some will be identified as corresponding to what they now know about their childhood. They look for mental pictures of the outside of the house, or the street where they lived. To remember childhood, however, it is necessary to go back inside the body. As a child, you never did have much of an image of what the outside of the house looked like, and the street, if you were to return, would bear little resemblance to your memories. What you will recall (and the process of recalling it is quite different from visual recall) will be the wet slop of a cloth on your face as you vainly turn your head this way and that trying to escape from firm hands holding your head. You will suddenly get a sensation of your vest being pulled off by competent, remorseless hands. You remember your childhood not with the objectivity of sight but with the subjectivity of the body itself.

4

Time, Space and Love

Spring 1984

Rapunzel Revisited   *31 March 1984*

We were listening again to the cassette of the story of Rapunzel. When
we came to the part where the witch throws the prince out of the window
of the tower on to the thorns which blind him, and where the prince
wanders through the forest with his stick looking for Rapunzel, Thomas
asked, 'Why was he blind?'

'Because his eyes were poorly,' I said, adding, 'My eyes are poorly.'

In a very serious and probing tone, he asked me, 'Are you blind?'

'Yes, I am,' I answered.

He turned towards me, and I sensed that he was examining me
closely. 'Your eyes are closed.'

I realized that this was true. Sometimes my eyes get very itchy and
watery, and I tend then to keep them closed. I opened my eyes wide,
and said, 'Yes, but even when I open my eyes, I still can't see, because
my eyes are poorly.'

'Can't you see the pictures?' he asked.

'No.'

'But I can see the pictures.'

'Your eyes aren't poorly,' I said.

I gently put my hand over his eyes, closing the lids and keeping them
firmly closed. 'Now can you see?' I said.

'No.'

I took my hand away. 'Now?'

'Yes, I can see now.'

68

'Your eyes aren't poorly,' I said. I repeated this some half-dozen times, and he seemed to enjoy it, but accepted it very quietly and thoughtfully. Again and again he repeated, 'Yes, my eyes aren't poorly. Yes, I can see,' each time I took my hand away.

We continued to listen to the story of Rapunzel, but a few moments later he interrupted again. 'When did you get blind?' he asked abruptly.

'It happened just a few days before you were born,' I said.

'What made your eyes go poorly?'

'They were sick,' I said, 'and the doctors couldn't make them better.' We continued with the story.

This was a very serious and important exchange. For the first time having poorly eyes, being blind, not being able to see, not being able to see pictures, were all associated. It is realized now that this constitutes a difference between me and Thomas, and that it is part of my own personal life-history.

The Rapunzel story is quite important in children's understanding of blindness, or their misunderstanding of it. I remember being in Wales on a summer holiday in 1981. Imogen, then aged eight, asked me, 'Daddy, if I cried and the tears fell on your eyes, would you be able to see again?' I am sure that she had picked this idea up from Rapunzel, for this is how the story ends.

Less Space, More Time   *17 April 1984*

Michael tells me that he thinks my perception of time has undergone a change since I lost my sight. He thinks that of all the people in the Faculty I am the only one who always seems to have plenty of time. Everyone else is rushing around, chasing their tails, trying to cram every minute with necessary tasks and to squeeze the last drop out of time. I alone seem to have all the time in the world. Michael remarked that in my work I don't cut corners; I just go on, doing what has to be done, until it is finished. It does not matter how much time it takes. In his own work, he has to cut corners all day long, in order to get his work finished.

Michael suggests that this different attitude to time, or position within time, may be partly due to the fact that I am not under pressure from another life. I do not have to leave the office at 5 p.m. in order to catch the garage so that I can get the car home so my wife can use it tonight. I do not have to get to the supermarket before it closes. There is a sense in which other people are not dependent upon my time.

Michael also wonders whether the fact that I cannot see the change in the day as the evening draws on is a factor. I press my clock. It says

69

that the time is 5.45 p.m. This is an abstract measure of time. It is a fact, spoken by a synthetic voice. I do not perceive the rise and decline of the day.

I think there is much truth in all this. Sighted people can bend time. For sighted people, time is sometimes slow and sometimes rapid. They can make up for being lazy by rushing later on. Things can be gathered up quickly in a few minutes. It is a bit like the change in your sense of time when you buy a car. Journeys that previously took two hours now take twenty minutes. You are amazed at how much more you can squeeze in. In this way, you force time to your will. Time, for sighted people, is that against which they fight.

For me, as a blind person, time is simply the medium of my activities. It is that inexorable context within which I do what must be done. For example, the reason why I do not seem to be in a hurry as I go around the building is not that I have less to do than my colleagues, but I am simply unable to hurry. It takes me almost exactly twenty-two minutes to walk from my front door to my office. I cannot do it in fifteen minutes, and if I tried to take thirty minutes over it, I would probably get lost, because knowledge of the route depends, to some extent, upon maintaining the same speed. The measured pace, the calm concentration, the continual recollection of exactly how far one has come and how far is still to go, the pause at each marked spot to make sure that one is orientated, all this must be conducted at the same controlled pace. Whether it rains or shines, I just go on.

It is also a matter of what one expects to be able to wrench out of time. When I had sight, I would have worked with feverish haste, correcting forty footnotes in a single morning. Now, I am happy if, with the help of a sighted reader, by the end of the morning I have corrected ten. I do not think to myself, 'Oh damn. I've only done ten.' I think, 'Good. That's ten done. Only another three mornings like this and the job will be finished.' I am so glad that I am able to do it at all. The simplicity, the careful planning, the long-term preparation, the deliberateness with which the blind person must live, all this means that he cannot take advantage of time by suddenly harvesting a whole lot of it.

Perhaps all severe disabilities lead to a decrease in space and an increase in time. I think of my friend Chris with his multiple sclerosis. Without his mobility machine, his range is about twenty yards. With the machine, which travels at about four miles an hour, his space is extended. He can rove for eight or twelve miles and come home again. Nevertheless, his space has shrunk relatively to what it was when he was in normal health. Time, on the other hand, has strangely expanded. It takes him forty-five minutes to tie up his shoelaces in the morning. It doesn't matter. He does not get impatient. He just does it. That is how long it takes to tie shoelaces. I think of Clive Inman, with his back injuries, lying in the Stoke Mandeville bed in the spinal unit at the Hexham Hospital. Space to him is diminished to the size of his bed. On the other hand, for those twelve long weeks, he has all the time in the world. He can lie there all day, spend hours talking to friends, listening to radio, thinking. It no longer matters if it takes five minutes careful concentration to pick something up.

When you have a lot of time, you experience time-inflation. The price of each hour goes up, because of the cost involved in the performance of each tiny task, but because the tasks are long and take so many hours the distinct value of each hour seems to deteriorate. The increasing cost is associated with a decreasing value. The hours become cheap in contrast to the necessary tasks which must be accommodated within them. You are no longer fighting against the clock but against the task. You no longer think of the time it takes. You only think of what you have to do. It cannot be done any faster. Time, against which you previously fought, becomes simply the stream of consciousness within which you act. For the deaf-blind person, space is confined to his body, but he has lots of time.

Modern technology seeks to expand human space and compress human time. The disabled person, on the other hand, finds that space is contracted and time is expanded. It is because of the space-time co-ordinates within which the blind person lives that his or her life becomes gradually different from the lives of sighted people, particularly in a time of high technology.

Acoustic Space   *27 April 1984*

What is the world of sound? I have been spending some time out of doors trying to respond to the special nature of the acoustic world. I am impressed by the many different aspects of reality, the range and depth of the contact points between myself and something created by sound.

The tangible world sets up only as many points of reality as can be touched by my body, and this seems to be restricted to one problem at a time. I can explore the splinters on the park bench with the tip of my finger but I cannot, at the same time, concentrate upon exploring the pebbles with my big toe. I can use all ten fingers when I am exploring the shape of something but it is quite difficult to explore two objects simultaneously, one with each hand. It is true that, if many people were poking me, I would feel all the prods with various parts of my body but this would not tell me very much about the world, only about my body.

The world revealed by sound is so different. It is true that I cannot listen to two different tape-recorded books at the same time, but that has to do with speech. I am thinking of the way in which sound places one within a world.

On Holy Saturday I sat in Cannon Hill Park while the children were playing. I heard the footsteps of passers-by, many different kinds of footsteps. There was the flip-flop of sandals and the sharper, more delicate sound of high-heeled shoes. There were groups of people walking together with different strides creating a sort of patter, being overtaken now by one, firm, long stride, or by the rapid pad of a jogger. There were children, running along in little bursts, and stopping to get on and off squeaky tricycles or scooters. The footsteps came from both sides. They met, mingled, separated again. From the next bench, there was the rustle of a newspaper and the murmur of conversation. Further out, to the right and behind me, there was the car park. Cars were stopping and starting, arriving and departing, doors were being slammed. Far over to the left, there was the main road. I heard the steady, deep roar of the through traffic, the buses and the trucks. In front of me was the lake. It was full of wildfowl. The ducks were quacking, the geese honking, and other birds which I could not identify were calling and cranking. There was continual flapping of wings, splashing and squabbling, as birds took off and landed on the surface, or fought over scraps of bread. There was the splash of the paddle boats, the cries of the children, and the bump as two boats collided. Parents on shore called out encouragement or warning. Further away, from the larger expanse of the lake, there was the different sound of the rowing boats as they swished past, and beyond that was the park. People were playing football. I heard the shouting, running feet, the impact of leather upon leather as the ball was kicked. There seemed to be several groups playing different games. Here there were boys; further over in that direction there seemed to be a group of young children playing. Over this whole scene, there was the wind. The trees behind me were murmuring, the shrubs and bushes along the side of the paths rustled, leaves and scraps of paper were blown along the path. I leant back and drank it all in. It was an astonishingly varied and rich panorama of movement, music and information. It was absorbing and fascinating.

The strange thing about it, however, is that it was a world of nothing but action. Every sound was a point of activity. Where nothing was happening, there was silence. That little part of the world then died, disappeared. The ducks were silent. Had they gone or was something holding their rapt attention? The boat came to rest. Were people leaning on the oars, or had they tied it to the edge and gone away? Nobody was walking past me just now. This meant that the footpath itself had disappeared. I could only remind myself of its direction by considering that it ran parallel to the bench upon which I sat. Even the traffic on the main road had paused. Were the lights red? When there is rest, everything else passes out of existence. To rest is not to be. To do is to be. Mine is not a world of being; it is a world of becoming. The world of being, the silent, still world where things simply are, that does not exist. The rockery, the pavilion, the skyline of high-rise flats, the flagpoles over the cricket ground, none of this is really there. The world of happenings, of movement and conflict, that is there.

The acoustic world is one in which things pass in and out of existence. This happens with such surprising rapidity. There seems to be no intermediate zone of approach. There is a sudden cry from the lake, 'Hello Daddy!'; my children are there in their paddle boat. Previously, a moment ago, they were not there. Not until they greeted me with a cry could I distinguish them from the rest of the background sounds. There was no gradual approach. While the world which greets me in this way is active, I am passive. I cannot stop these stimulations flooding me. I just sit here. The creatures emitting the noise have to engage in some activity. They have to scrape, bang, hit, club, strike surface upon surface, impact, make their vocal chords vibrate. They must take the initiative in announcing their presence to me. For my part, I have no power to explore them. I cannot penetrate them or discover them without their active co-operation. They must utter their voice, their sound. It is thus a world which comes to me, which springs into life for me, which has no existence apart from its life towards me.

The intermittent nature of the acoustic world is one of its most striking features. In contrast, the perceived world is stable and continuous. The seen world cannot escape from your eyes. Even in the darkness, you can use a torch and force things into visibility, but I have only very limited power over the acoustic world.

Here is another feature of the acoustic world: it stays the same whichever way I turn my head. This is not true of the perceptible world. It changes as I turn my head. New things come into view. The view looking that way is quite different from the view looking this way. It is not like that with sound. New noises do not come to my attention as I turn my head around. I may allow my head to hang limply down upon my chest; I may lean right back and face the sky. It makes little difference.

Perhaps there is some slight shading of quality, but the acoustic world is mainly independent of my movement. This heightens the sense of passivity. Instead of me having to search things out and uncover fresh portions of my world by my own effort as I fix my gaze first here then there, in the acoustic world there is something which is rather indifferent to my attempts to penetrate it. This is a world which I cannot shut out, which goes on all around me, and which gets on with its own life. I can, of course, train myself to pay attention to it; I can learn to distinguish this from that sound, become more practised in judging distance and so on. Nevertheless, my ears remain fixed in a stationary head, while my eyes, if I could see, would be darting here and there with innumerable movements in a head which itself was moving.

Acoustic space is a world of revelation.

Making Love in the Pub   *1 May 1984*

Last night I dreamt that I was in a pub. Marilyn and I were making love. The scene changed to the crowded bar. An announcement was heard over the public address system. 'Will the blind man at the bar please report immediately because his wife and daughter have been involved in an accident.' The notice was repeated. In the dream I now had an image of myself, holding the white cane, hearing the notice, stupefied with anxiety. A second time the notice was twice repeated. Then I was at the back door of the pub. At the end of the drive there was a car. Marilyn and Imogen were in it. I couldn't get to them fast enough. A scream broke from my lips. 'Meg! Immy!' Then, whether with assistance or not I cannot tell, I was at the car. Everything was all right. It had been a false alarm. Imogen was fine. Marilyn was fine. I told them about the announcement in the bar, but everything was OK.

In this dream I hear myself described as a blind man, I see myself holding a stick, I once again sense the panic of not being able to get quickly enough to loved ones in distress. In the dream, however, it is not clear whether I am led or conducted. I seem to be able to get there by myself.

The main subject of the dream is fear of losing Marilyn through blindness. This seems to be corrected by the later realization that, after all, this will not happen. So my dream says.

This is a dream about blindness as well as a blind person's dream.

'Don't You Want Your Sight Back?'   *8 May 1984*

Last Thursday one of my friends was driving me home from a meeting. I asked her if she would mind if I collected a meal from an Indian takeaway. We parked on the double yellow lines outside one of the restaurants in Bristol Street. My friend helped me as far as the door of the restaurant, where we were met by an affable man who seemed to be a person of authority in the place. My friend returned to her parked car and I was escorted to a table. My escort introduced himself to me as an entertainer who worked every evening in the restaurant. His name was, he said, Benito Luigi, not an Indian, but a Sicilian. He explained that, although in his capacity as an entertainer, a magician and a conjuror, he worked in the restaurant, his essential work was as a hypnotherapist.

He asked me if my companion would like to come inside and have a cup of coffee, and offered me coffee too. He would keep an eye out for the police, and would explain the situation should the need arise. He called my friend from her car and we were both served with coffee. He entertained her by describing his business and his specialities.

Turning to me, he asked if I would mind answering some personal questions. I knew now what was coming, and was ready for it. He asked if I was completely blind, how long I had been blind, the cause of my blindness and whether I was completely satisfied that nothing more could be done. He told me candidly that there was only one thing I could now have hope in, and that was my own willpower. My sight depended upon my will, and he, through hypnotherapy, could restore and strengthen my will.

I asked Luigi whether he could restore a limb which had been lost during a road accident. He said 'No,' I pointed out that my eyes were a bit like that. This seemed to give him pause for thought. He hesitated. 'You got no eyes? They gone?' I took my glasses off and showed him my left eye, which is completely white. I told him that that was not really a normal eye. Significant components had been removed or destroyed. I told him that the lenses from my eyes were gone and that the retina in both eyes had long since perished. Willpower could not restore these physical structures any more than willpower could make a new arm grow.

Nothing daunted, Luigi told me about some of the marvellous cures he had performed, including terminal cancer. 'You're not a hypnothera-pist. You're a faith healer!' I told him. He appealed to my companion for her opinion of the case. She was inclined to agree with me. This did not seem like a case of weakened will but a case of structural defect. Perhaps seeing that our food was about to be brought to the table, Luigi made one final attempt. 'But all you need is willpower! Don't you have willpower? Don't you *want* your sight back?'

'Of course I want my sight back,' I said, laughing at the joke. 'But, on the other hand, don't misunderstand me. I am a contented person.'

He replied, 'I see that you are contented. Yes, I see that you laugh a lot, you are a happy man. Nevertheless, you must want your sight back.'

I agreed, and at that moment our food arrived. Luigi gave me his business card, and we bid each other friendly farewells.

On the way home in the car, my friend and I discussed this amusing incident. She was delighted by this new acquaintance, and amused by his vivacity and his charm. She was rather intrigued at the thought of being hypnotized by him, and wondered what it would be like. When we stopped outside the house, she asked in a hesitant but curious tone, 'But, John, what about yourself? Why did you not accept? What harm could it do? Do you think you have got to the point where you really don't want your sight back?'

I was taken aback at this, and replied, 'How can you say that? Of course I want my sight back! I will never accept the loss of my sight!'

'But, John,' she said, 'you do seem so well adjusted to it. You always seem to be so poised, so happy, you seem to function so well.'

'You don't know half the truth,' I said warmly. 'I will never accept the human losses involved in blindness, and I will never accept futile help from that sort of quarter either. Don't you see that I would find it even more degrading, more humiliating, that it would only be to betray any courage and dignity which I may have left? There are some situations in life when you have to carry out a protracted but dignified warfare against despair and not allow yourself to be made the emotional slave of those who offer false hopes.'

This line of argument had little impact. My loyal and affectionate friend was still inclined to think that it must be a combination of pride and complacency which held me back from accepting such a harmless offer. For my part, to persist with the military metaphor, if blindness is going to vanquish me, I would rather be found dead with the wounds on my chest and not in my back.

Sin: The Cause of Blindness   9 May 1984

At church last Sunday, we again met our faith-healing friend, Mr Cresswell. Perhaps my attitude had hardened somewhat in the meantime, partly because of the encounter with the hypnotherapist in the Indian restaurant and partly because Marilyn had made me have a couple of spoonfuls of cod liver oil mixed with honey, and had been mildly disapproving when I refused any more.

Mr Cresswell came up in a breezy manner, shook me by the hand, and asked me how things were. It was apparent that he was not very

Plymouth University
The Charles Seale-Hayne Library

Customer ID: *****11511

Title: On sight & insight : a journey
into the world of blindness /
ID: 9004769314
Due: 25/03/2016 23:59:00 GMT

Total items: 1
12 Feb 2016
Checked out: 1
Overdue: 0
Hold requests: 0

Due date of borrowed items subject
to change. Please check your
University email regularly for recall
notices to avoid incurring a fine.

Thank you for using the
3M SelfCheck™ System.

Plymouth University
The Charles Seale-Hayne Library

Customer ID: *****1511

Title: On sight & insight : a journey
into the world of blindness /
ID: 9004769314
Due: 25/03/2016 23:59:00 GMT

Total items: 1
12 Feb 2016
Checked out: 1
Overdue: 0
Hold requests: 0

Due date of borrowed items subject
to change. Please check your
University email regularly for recall
notices to avoid incurring a fine

Thank you for using the
3M SelfCheck™ System.

interested in how things were, since I suppose the white cane I was holding told its own story, but he apologized for not having visited us again, and then announced that he had a word from the Lord for me. The message was that the Lord was instructing me to get hold of a small Bible and carry it always in my pocket. From now on, I must always have the word of God with me, it must go with me, this is what God had said: 'Let the word go with you.'

'I'm sorry, Mr Cresswell,' I said, 'but I am not prepared to do that. I have a lot of things to put in my pockets and I am not prepared to clutter them up with one more thing. I carry the word of God always in my head and in my heart, and I see no point in carrying it in my pocket as well.'

Mr Cresswell waxed rather eloquent at this, and told me roundly that God was telling me the simple thing that I should now do in order to have my sight back and if I were not prepared to obey him then I should not be surprised if my sight were not restored. Sin was the cause of blindness, as of all illness, and sin lay in the resistance and pride of men in refusing to obey the word of God, and to do the simple things God said.

'Mr Cresswell,' I said, 'I see that we have very different ideas about God, and about sin and about sight. I do not accept any of your ideas about these things. Whether we live or die, we are always the Lord's and I am not prepared to be put under emotional pressure to do all these strange things week by week. You are advising me to accept magical, superstitious practices.'

'No, no,' he expostulated, 'these are the words of the Lord!'

He pursued me down the aisle, as Marilyn and I began to make our way to the door, warning me that I was treading a very dangerous path, and that I would not find healing that way.

As we got into the car, I felt slightly regretful that I had, perhaps, alienated a kindly and well-meaning man through speaking the truth too directly, but on the other hand, as I remarked to Marilyn, I cannot allow myself to be blackmailed into doing all sorts of nonsensical things through weakly capitulating to futile hopes.

'You Bastard, You're not Blind' *11 May 1984*

I was walking home after an evening class. It was a little after eight o'clock. There was not much movement around the campus. I heard running feet approaching, stopping perhaps twenty yards away. A fierce, harsh, male voice, distorted with anger and malice, shouted, 'Are you blind, mate? You're not blind! How did you get blind? You're not blind!'

I was so surprised, both by the abruptness and the manner of this address, that I stood perfectly still. I waited for a moment, in silence, wondering whether to reply. Again my accuser spat out his question, 'Are you blind?'

Quietly, but hoping that my voice sounded firm and clear, I replied, 'Yes, I am blind.'

I sensed that he was coming closer to me. 'You dirty fucking bastard! You're not blind! How did you get blind? You're not blind!'

'No,' I replied, 'you are wrong. I am blind.'

I tried to resist the impulse to lift up my briefcase and hold it in front of me, for I had the impression that he was about to attack me, to punch me, to see whether I was blind or not. Perhaps he would see whether or not I would try to duck. I resisted the temptation, however, and stayed quite still, looking in his direction, since I thought that any sign of nervousness might have encouraged him to attack me. He seemed to move off to the left a little, and when he spoke again it was from further away. Again he shouted in the same tone of malicious anger and hatred, 'You're not blind! How did you get blind?' From even further away, he sent after me one final 'You're not blind!' and then he seemed to disappear.

I was, rather naturally, a little hesitant about proceeding on my route. What if he had come back and was standing only a few feet in front of me? I waited a few more moments to see if he would shout out again. I then realized that there was a car parked on the far side of the road along which I was walking. I got the impression that the driver had got out of his car during this incident, but was not getting back in. I heard him mutter to the person he was with, 'Silly bugger! What's he want to talk like that to him for?'

I took it that he was referring to my assailant, rather than to me, and was encouraged to call out, 'Is he gone?'

The driver asked me which way I was going. I misunderstood him, thinking that he was about to offer me a lift. 'Oh, it's all right,' I said. 'I can manage, thank you very much. I was just a bit startled, that's all.'

'No, which way are you going?' he asked again.

'I'm going straight ahead, down to the Bristol Road.'

'Oh, you're all right. He's gone off in the opposite direction.'

'Who was he?' I asked.

'I don't know.'

'What was he like? Was he drunk or something?'

'Don't know, couldn't tell.'

I thanked the driver for his help and went on my way.

Two or three years ago, when I still had a little residual vision, I was walking through the Selly Oak shops one night when, crossing a side street, a chap a few paces behind me shouted 'Look out, mate! There's a car! Stop!' I stopped rather sharply, startled because I had not heard anything coming. I took a step back towards the pavement from which I had come. A second voice spoke. 'It's all right mate, he's only kidding. You're all right to cross.' I did not look around or make any gesture of acknowledgement or thanks, but resumed my path across the road with what I hoped was a distant dignity. These were simply young fellows having a bit of fun. The man on the campus was rather more strange. A blind friend who makes a living by busking in shopping centres told me that he is often attacked by youths who accuse him of being a fraud. I have never had this particular experience before.

In School
13 May 1984

I spent the whole day teaching in a nearby comprehensive school. The head of the religious education department picked me up from my home in his car in the morning. Most of the time, I was with him, joining in from time to time, but one class I taught entirely alone. I had been wondering how I would handle the questioning and the discussion, so important in religious education. Having introduced me, the class teacher asked the pupils to raise their hands in the normal way and he himself would call upon one of them to answer my question. As it happened, this was unnecessary. Lots of hands went up at my first question. I realized that when the children put their hands up, their clothes rustled, there was a slight in-drawing of breath, and if they were really enthusiastic, they would say 'S-s-s . . .', that being the first sound in the word 'sir'. The children may have been unaware of these sounds, but in a fairly quiet classroom, they provided enough guidance for me to point straight at a child with his or her hand up.

The class teacher told me that the first time I did this, the face of the child to whom I pointed was a picture of surprise. At the end of the double lesson, the same boy said to me, 'How did you know I was here?' It turned out that he was referring to his very first question of the afternoon. He had been amazed that I had pointed straight at him. When I explained to the class how I had been doing this, they were still amazed.

When the lesson was over, I remarked to the class teacher that I had been bluffing to some extent. I knew that most of the time there were many hands raised, and it was enough to point vaguely around to make sure that I was pointing at someone.

The teacher said that if this was the case, it was not obvious. Certainly, I seemed to waver slightly once or twice, but in the vast majority of cases, I was both pointing and looking at a child with her hand right up. This was an interesting discovery, and raised my confidence considerably.

I did have a problem, however, in that I had not anchored myself securely to a piece of furniture. I tended to wander slightly, and sometimes lost my sense of where the class was. I had to ask a general question of the whole class, so that I got the entire range of responses, and only then could I reorientate myself towards the angle of the classroom. Stepping back to regain contact with my chair once or twice, I found that I had drifted two or three feet from it. It is hard not to appear to fumble when trying to rediscover a chair like this in public. One of the lessons I have learned, then, is to position myself firmly, perhaps with a finger on a desk.

Do People Look Like Something?   *26 May 1984*

Marilyn described what somebody looked like. So and so had glasses and a beard, his hair and complexion were of a certain colour and shade, his features were pointed or rounded, his posture was tall but stooping, or he was rather thin, or whatever. I realized that these are all characteristics which I hardly ever think about. They are a category of missing items in my appraisal of people. I form some kind of general image of people, it is true. It does make a difference to me if I encounter a delicately manicured hand or a huge hairy fist. Similarly, when someone is leading me, and I place a finger under his or her elbow, I occasionally seize the opportunity of touching the forearm, and it does make a difference to my mental image of the person if the arm is thin and bony, or huge, and rounded like a barrel. These traces give me some suggestion of the general figure or dimensions of the person I am dealing with, and there is also the height from which the person's voice seems to be coming. But the intense anxiety which I used to feel about what people looked like during the early years of my blindness seems to have faded. The vivid experience of a series of projected images of the person's face flashing through my imagination as I talk with him or her has gone completely.

What is now of supreme importance to me is the voice, and what I can perhaps describe as 'personal magnetism'. I think this is now true even in my relationships with women. The importance of the beauty of the face has diminished. In speaking engagements, I am not as troubled by the absence of visual feedback as I used to be, although I do find it helpful to provoke some kind of aural feedback, such as shuffling, laughter, questions and so on.

In general, whether with crowds or with individuals, I depend more and more upon my awareness of a kind of receptivity. In a poor auditorium, you are conscious of the music from the orchestra fighting its way towards you, whereas in a well-designed concert hall, the sound is presented to you in its immediacy and freshness. So it is with an audience. I believe that I can feel when an audience is not understanding me. In contrast, there is a kind of openness, a quality of attention, when I am being received with understanding and sympathy. Many sighted public speakers also feel this kind of response in an audience, but I am not sure what the cues are for the blind public speaker. Perhaps it is a matter of the warmth of the first reception, or maybe it has to do with one's confidence in one's own material, knowing that it has been well prepared and presented. At any rate, what people look like no longer matters.

Blindness in Eastern and Western Religions
9 June 1984

Generally speaking, blind people have a bad time in religion. Almost all religions, ancient and modern, regard any form of physical disability as a sign of sinfulness. This may be thought of in magical terms, or it may be expressed in ritual as, for example, when a disabled person is not permitted to be a priest or to offer a sacrifice. Worst of all, it may take an ethical form. In that case, the disabled person is thought to have committed a sin, whether in the present life or in some former life, or to be under some kind of divine or providential punishment or disgrace.

There may, however, be differences between the spiritualities of the East and the West, and these may affect the situation of disabled, particularly blind, people. In the West, the Jewish/Christian tradition has tended to emphasize the active life. The believer is called to change the world. The grace of God is seen at work in such activity, in redeeming the world and in bringing in God's kingdom.

In the great religions of Asia, particularly Hinduism and Buddhism, the emphasis is perhaps more on inwardness. There may be a renunciation of the world in some sense; the world may be regarded as a form of divine play, as being a lesser reality from which the believer is to gradually move towards a greater reality. Whereas the Western form tends to lead to heroic saintliness, the Eastern type encourages meditative or contemplative saintliness.

In Asian religions, blind people are often respected as possessing one of the keys to inwardness, but in the West the disabled person is sometimes seen as being less fully and actively an agent of God's salvation, simply because disability has imposed a less obviously active life. The blindness which in India helps one on the road to holiness is thought of as a hindrance in Europe.

The Protestant tradition of Christianity presents a special problem. Here, the desire to become an instrument of God is often particularly strong. Moreover, the emphasis upon the Word of God means that the deaf (who cannot hear the words) and the blind (who cannot read print) are marginalized. In addition, there has been a tendency in Protestantism away from anything which would appeal to the other senses, such as bells which can be rung, statues which can be touched, incense which can be smelt. So it is that in Protestantism the disabled person, the one who cannot act, is often seen as part of the problem, rather than as being part of the answer. The presence of the disabled person becomes an offence to active faith.

In Roman Catholicism, disabled people go on pilgrimage to places of miracles such as Lourdes but if a miracle does not take place, there is no problem. People go to receive strength and courage; some receive healing, others do not. There is a tolerant acceptance of a variety of responses and outcomes. In the Protestant evangelical tradition it is sometimes not like this. Blind people who were noteworthy recipients of the healing power of Jesus, as reported in the Gospels, seem to present a particular problem. Many blind people report a strong pressure from such groups to accept miraculous healing. I have been told of persons who, having lost sight, felt obliged after a year or two of unceasing pressure, to find a new church in which to worship. Sometimes this pressure is so intense that one could speak of a Christian persecution of blind people.

Blindness is a form of brokenness, and the value of the broken life is recognized in both East and West. In Indian religious traditions, one breaks away from the secular life and enters a period of contemplation later in life. Sense perception may be broken in order to open inward sight. In the Western traditions, although activity in the service of God is valued highly, it is also recognized, especially in Christianity, that in the end this activity must be supported by the grace of God. In Protestantism, it is not being active but having faith that saves one. How does the brokenness of blindness relate to these different ideas?

The disabled person is broken as far as action in this world is concerned. He or she must depend upon the help of others to some extent; in that sense there is a living by grace. It may be, however, that many Western Christians somehow feel that disability lacks value because it has not been chosen. It is not the result of a voluntary submission of one's will to God, but is imposed by accident or illness. In the West it is not so easy to interpret the blind person as someone who has reached a certain point along a recognized spiritual path. Rather, the tendency is to think of the disabled person as someone who has been prevented, for some inscrutable reason, from setting out upon that path.

I spoke with some members of the Hare Krishna group who were having a meeting in Paradise Circus in Birmingham city centre. I was received with great courtesy and told that, as a blind person, I was already probably in a state of spiritual grace. I was told that the Hindu tradition venerates blindness because of the spiritual gifts which it can confer. Be that as it may, I have to say that I have never received such a reaction from any Christian group. At best, blindness is an obstacle to be overcome by courageous endurance, and at worst it is an opportunity for God to display his grace by banishing it through a healing miracle.

Am I a Workaholic? *17 June 1984*

What gives me this feeling of tension after several days away from work or from my office? It builds up into quite a strong sense of discomfort, anxiety and then depression. This becomes so disquieting that it is almost painful.

To some extent, I think it is the frustration caused by the presence of the children. In that situation, I become most keenly aware of blindness. Perhaps another factor is that any blind person is, to some extent, starved of information. I run short of facts. My brain demands something new to know.

I can be plunged quite suddenly into such feelings of deprivation through some little incident or other. As we were crossing the road from the car park to the entrance of the airport the other day, I called out, 'Is anybody holding Lizzie's hand?' In the rush to get over the road, the family simply ignored my question. This was perfectly sensible of them, since this was the moment to get safely to the footpath, not to start discussing who was holding whom. Nevertheless, I suddenly felt out of things, that my ability to watch over Lizzie had been destroyed, that there was no point in trying to care for her or bothering. What was the point,

I found myself wondering, in asking who is with her, what she is doing, and if she is safe? I was a mere lump of fat being carted around.

On the other hand, a few days ago I attended a conference in London where I found many people I knew. All day long I was meeting old friends, being introduced to new colleagues, catching up on bits of news about various events and finding out new developments in my work. I hardly had time to realize that I was blind, and the day passed by quickly.

What affects me is the cumulative experience of the inescapable presence of blindness. Perhaps it is also the lack of control, and this may well be why I find it so exhausting. It is in intellectual work that I find refreshment, partly because I can almost entirely forget that I am blind. The social demands of public life and the personal demands of family life seem to create so many situations in which I become not only aware but painfully aware of blindness. On the whole, however, such experiences are not as common nor as severe as they were six months ago.

An Empty Presence   *18 June 1984*

Sometimes, when I am entirely alone in the Education building, I have a strong sense of presence. As I go through the double glass doors into the foyer, I suddenly feel that it is alive, although the building is deserted. On a Sunday afternoon, or late at night, even strolling around at 5.15 on a quiet afternoon, the building feels empty. To check this impression, I can walk around the whole place and meet nobody. Even if there are a couple of people having a chat on one of the landings, it does not dispel the sense of emptiness, which is combined with the sense of presence.

Whenever there are people working in a large building like this, there must be fifty or sixty PCs and printers clicking away, doors being opened and closed, filing cabinet drawers sliding in and out and furniture being moved. All of this, together with the weight and the movements of the hundreds of people in the building, most of whom are talking, must set up a background of minute vibrations, both tactile and audible, of which one is barely aware, and yet which create a sense of life, of fullness, of being held in a human world. When the building is empty, a strange lifeless, static quality emerges.

This is true of the office block but not of my own home. I cannot tell whether the house is occupied or not when I come in. Everybody may be out on the back terrace, but the house does not feel particularly empty. In a carpeted house with fairly small rooms, the acoustic environment is quite different. It is the large, modern office block, with its long, tiled corridors, its lecture theatres and its stairwells that sets up this background of buzzing fullness.

But what about the sense of presence? Why does the building exercise presence when it has become empty? This must be to do with my awareness of facial vision or echo location.

It must be that when a familiar building is empty, I become more sharply aware of its many surfaces, its ceilings and walls, its recesses and corridors. Different angles, volumes and distances would be pressing against me as I turn around on the same spot. While actual sound does not change much as I turn around, this kind of strange physical sensation, even if it is based upon hearing, does change. It must be more than mere hearing; there must be a certain sensitivity of the entire body to vibrations and to air pressure as well as to inaudible echoes. It is because the entire body is involved that the result is this strange feeling of being surrounded by a presence. This would make me feel surveyed or observed. It is a bit like the feeling one sometimes has of being watched, except that it is as if the whole building is watching me, is aware of me, knows I am there. Now my imagination is surely running away with me.

Nevertheless, this is rather an eerie feeling. I cannot say that I particularly like it. I sometimes feel that I am bursting into the building against its will, and that it resists my intrusion. I fight back by singing and tramping noisily along, clicking my stick briskly on the steps. This seems to put the building in its place and lets it know who is in charge around here.

5

The Wind and the Sea

Summer 1984

Body-time

19 June 1984

If blind people live in time, deaf people live in space. Deaf people measure time by seeing movement. If, however, deaf people gaze out upon a world in which there is no movement, such as the stars, a deserted street, or some mountain scenery, then there is a quality of permanence, of static consistency. In losing this kind of awareness of space, blind people have less awareness of unchangeability. The world of blind people is more ephemeral, since sounds come and go.

Consider the importance of body-time to blind people. A deaf person walking home has no problems in timing the point at which he leaves the public footpath and enters his own house. His body is placed within a number of pictures of his environment which are fairly consistent from day to day. When a picture of a certain kind, the shape of his house, or the colour of his front gate appears before him, he knows which way to go. With blind people, this sense of being in a place is less pronounced.

Let us take an example of internal body timing. For several days recently, I have been overshooting my front gate by about fifteen yards, which would be about the length occupied by a single house. I could not work out why I was doing this, but I did it several times in a week. My house is about a hundred and fifty yards from the corner of the block. As I begin that final part of my walk home, I seem to know more or less how far I have to walk. I do not count the paces, I just know how much work I have to do in order to arrive. I am usually tapping the line of fences, and this gives me all sorts of clues about my exact position, but

86

even if I am being guided by somebody else and have no contact with the fences, I seem to know how far it is.

At present, the second house up from the corner is having a new roof, and the footpath is blocked with piles of roofing materials. It is clear that my body clock had been resetting itself again after that interruption, and then allowing me to go the expected distance. I was overshooting by about the same distance as that which was occupied by the tiles on the footpath. For the blind person, the house is only there because of past experience. Space is reduced to one's own body, and the position of the body is known not by what objects have been passed but by how long it has been in motion. Position is thus measured by time.

Let us take another example. A page of a printed book is an area of space. When you are reading with your eyes you traverse this space until it is all covered, and then turning the page you encounter another space and so on. The same is true of braille. Books recorded on tape are, however, like speech itself, always moving, and measured by time. We may say that the problem for the blind author not using braille is to find an equivalent in time for everything which the sighted author does in space.

This brings us to the difference in the blind perception of people. For the deaf person, people have an abiding presence. They are there, all the time, every day. For a blind person, people are not there unless they speak. Many times I have continued a conversation with a sighted friend, only to discover that he was not there. He may have walked away without telling me. He may have nodded or smiled, thinking the conversation was over. From my point of view, he has suddenly vanished.

When you are blind, a hand suddenly grabs you. A voice suddenly addresses you. There is no anticipation or preparation. There is no hiding around the corner. There is no lying low. I *am* grasped. I *am* greeted. I am passive in the presence of that which accosts me. I cannot escape it. Normal people can choose whom they want to speak to, as they wander around the streets or the market-place. People are already there for the sighted person; they have a presence prior to their being greeted, and the sighted person can choose whether or not to turn that presence into a relationship by addressing an acquaintance. For the blind person, people are in motion, they are temporal, they come and they go. They come out of nothing; they disappear. St Augustine has a parable about the human soul. He says it is like a bird which bursts into a large building, flutters for a while, and then finds an escape and disappears. This idea of being visited, of being blessed by receiving a visitation, seems to me to be quite important in the blind experience of other people.

A Novel Experience   *22 June 1984*

I am impressed by the similarity between the experience of being blind and the experience of getting to know a world as described by a novelist. When you read that a certain character went into a room, and that it was furnished in such and such a way, with pictures on the walls and a window looking out over the bay, it is just like the blind experience of being shown into a room by a sighted person. A blind person can verify most of what he or she is told about a room, and to that extent has the advantage over the sighted novel reader.

On the other hand, if the description is of the outside of a building, or of scenery, then as a blind person I do not have any advantage over the sighted reader. I know no more than the author chooses to tell me. One might say that a novelist is describing things which have no real existence, whereas the sighted person is telling me about things which he or she, at least, can see. One sighted person, however, will see something quite differently from another, and I will often be given descriptions of the same place which have very little in common. That increases my feeling of being in a novel, because I am experiencing the world through the imagination of others.

This is heightened by the fact that I read novels on cassette. Someone is talking to me, whether it is the guide conducting me around the cathedral, or the novelist describing a cathedral. It is all talk. For the sighted person, on the other hand, there is a clear difference between what is read and what is heard.

The blind person's experience of life is so often second hand. A novelist tells you that one of the characters gave an ironic smile. One of my sighted friends tells me that so and so gave an ironic smile. In neither case can I verify it. Beards and glasses can be felt, but not ironic smiles. Sometimes I ask another sighted friend to comment on the same situation. I get such different replies that it makes me rather sceptical. Did she look rather tired last night or not? Was he smiling ironically or sympathetically? My lack of independence in forming these judgements leads me into scepticism.

For blind people, much of the experience of life takes on a literary quality. It becomes a story book. I do not so much live life as have life told to me.

Naming   *3 July 1984*

I have just returned from a conference in Ontario. I made a big effort in getting to know all of the eighty or so people there. If I heard someone speaking in one of the public sessions, and could not recognize the voice, I would whisper to the person next to me, asking who it was. I was surprised by the number of times my neighbours were unable to reply. They recognized the speaker; they knew it was the person with whom they had had such and such a conversation, but they did not know the name. Even late in the conference, when I would have thought that most people had got to know each other, I found that if I asked an acquaintance to take me over to anyone in the room whose name he knew, there might be no more than two or three in a room with twenty people in it whose names were familiar. I discussed this with a colleague, pointing out that it was relatively easy for a sighted person to get to know a group of seventy or eighty people, whereas a blind person had to work hard at it. My colleague replied that my assumptions about how sighted people got to know each other were mistaken. They do not, on the whole, get to know each other by name. That is part of it, of course, but it is more a requirement of courtesy. Sighted people get to know each other by recognizing each other's appearance, and all the things the new acquaintance has said and done are associated with that image of what he or she looks like. The appearance, the look of the person, is that around which all of the other items cluster. The name of the person is one additional item of information, but the appearance is that central core around which everything gathers.

For me, knowing someone hangs upon knowing the name. It is the same with streets. Sighted people often do not know the names of the streets they use every day. For the blind person, the name of the street is essential, so that one can ask where one is.

The name of a person, however, does not tell you much about what to expect. You can tell the sex, and often the nationality, and sometimes you might be able to make a rough guess at the age of the person. From the appearance of somebody, on the other hand, you can learn much more.

In Ontario, I worked by getting to know people's names. I had the list of names read to me again and again, and I could simply ask to be taken to somebody by name, and could keep on asking, until I met somebody who could do this. I kept on working down the list, name by name. Not until I heard the voice and felt the hand clasp which would, from now on, be associated with that name, did I form much of an expectation. Around the name I would build up the story of that person. The name is the verbal cue around which that particular story hangs.

When a blind person and a sighted person are making friends, it is a bit like the difference between the parables about the merchant who, having discovered a pearl of great price, sold everything he had to buy that pearl, and the one about the farmer, ploughing in the field, who accidentally discovered a hidden treasure. The sighted person, having formed an image of the pearl that was sought, takes steps to deepen that friendship. The blind person suddenly strikes treasure in the field. Without anticipation, without previous images, he or she encounters someone, enters into dialogue, and meets a surprising new story.

The people in the group around are not present to the blind person as if stretched out in space, as so many patches of colour, but they do have depths. They are like voices suspended upon stilts – a present emerging out of a past, in time rather than in space. Sight enables one to take a cross-section through somebody's life at the present moment. The blind person, however, takes a longitudinal section, back through time. This is not only a longer view of a person's life, but it takes longer to acquire.

Litmus Paper   4 July 1984

One of the most difficult aspects of blindness is the way it tends to make you passive in getting to know people. Not to be able to choose freely whom you want to speak with, not to be able to get to know somebody better by making a special point of greeting him or her: this problem has always worried me since I lost my sight.

I have been developing techniques to deal with this. I hope that these will restore to me some of the initiative in making and keeping human friendships.

Suppose I am talking with somebody after a meeting. How do I change partners? The sighted person has many little devices available. She can say, 'Oh, excuse me a minute, I just want to have a word with so and so.' The blind person cannot do this, because she has no easy way of knowing that so and so is over there. The sighted person can say, 'I'll be back in a minute. I'm just going to get another drink.' Not only have I found it very difficult to break away from a conversation, but my sighted friend finds it difficult to get away from me. He feels responsible for me. He cannot just go off and leave me standing there. It is an impasse. How can we get away from each other?

When I have decided that the time has come to stop talking to someone, I simply ask him or her to have a look around the room and to take me to someone else. Knowing the names of the people I want to speak to is, of course, all important. I may say, 'Well, I'm going to go and talk to somebody else now. Can you see if so and so is around?' This is not too good. It takes my friend ages to look around for a particular person. If my friend does not know this person, or if the person turns out not to be around, I am stuck. I find it better to ask, 'Can you see anybody at all you know?' Usually, my friend will say, 'Well, there's old so and so over there.' I say, 'Will you please take me to him and introduce me?' I repeat this process again and again. In this way I may manage to speak to a dozen people during the course of a fifteen-minute coffee break. I am also meeting new people, because my friends are introducing me to the people *they* know.

This technique works best in a meeting of a fairly regular group of people like a society or a church. It works well in a confined social situation like a conference where people are wearing name badges, or where everybody in the building is taking part in the same event, but the technique does have various problems. It makes it rather difficult for somebody who wants to talk to me to get a word in. Since I always appear to be in conversation, there are never the natural social spaces during which it is normally possible to intervene. Many people do not find it easy to adopt the direct approach: 'Excuse me, I'll just have a word with John now, if you don't mind.'

One of the interesting features of this technique is the enormous differences I find in the skill with which people seem to realize what it is I want, and are able to carry it out smoothly. Sometimes my conversational partner will embarrass me by shouting out, 'Excuse me, Bill! John Hull would like to have a word with you.'

Bill then breaks away from whoever he is with, comes over to me and says, 'Yes, John, what is it?' The truth is that I have nothing in particular to say to Bill. I merely wanted to shake hands with him and ask him how he is. The fact that the technique itself is so deliberate makes people think that I am deliberate in wanting to speak to the named individual. Other people seem to have a natural instinct for helping. They cannot only rattle off half a dozen names in quick succession, but can slide me into the new conversation in an unobtrusive way. I seem to have discovered a sort of litmus-paper test, a kind of social examination, which enables me to find out certain things about my new acquaintances quite quickly and, often, quite reliably.

It's awful, having to make such demands upon people all the time. The alternative, however, seems to be almost complete social marginalization and passivity.

Walking Together   *6 July 1984*

When I am walking into work, it is not unusual for people to ask if I need any help. Now, the truth is that on this route I do not need help. Usually,

I say, 'Thank you very much. I'm quite OK. I come along here every day. Thanks just the same for your offer.'

I am always grateful for these offers, since I am conscious of the fact that on an unfamiliar route I would probably be quite glad of some help. The sighted pedestrian, meeting me, may not know whether I am on one of my familiar routes or not.

Sometimes, the person who offers to help me is known to me already. It may be a neighbour, somebody who works in some other part of the University, or somebody who walked in with me on some earlier occasion. Usually I respond by saying, 'I don't need any help because this is one of my routes, but I am glad of your company and would like to walk along with you.'

Now, with me, a curious thing takes place. I lose my independence as soon as I accept my friend's company. This is because I must put a finger under the elbow of my companion, in order to locate him, to keep abreast of him, so as not to keep walking into him. I am like a hitch-hiker. I am being towed, moving more rapidly than would normally be possible.

Instead of waving my stick from side to side in front of me, I am either holding it steadily in front, just as a protection in case my friend forgets to tell me there is a lamppost, or I may have folded it up under my arm. Moreover, we have to have conversation. If you are walking along with somebody for company, you talk. This means that I cannot devote to my route the concentration which it would normally require.

When I am walking along this, my most familiar route, I have in my mind a screen with a sort of map of the area, and my own presence, like a pinpoint of light, moving along it. I continually refer to this to check up on my position. Here I am, coming along this portion of my route, having crossed the road, being about to cross that road, knowing that around the next corner there will be the traffic lights. I must never forget my position. That would be as if the light went out. I am continually verifying my position on this map by taking into account all sorts of little, familiar features. On this corner, the kerb is slightly higher. The curvature of the footpath is slightly more pronounced at this point. The road surface here is not quite the same as it was there. Here comes that little smooth patch. There are certain points along my route where I actually have to count the steps in order to avoid the lampposts. All of this requires constant attention. If I allow my concentration to lapse for a moment, I may get slightly out of position, I might walk into something, I might stray on to a busy road. I cannot do any of this and have a conversation at the same time.

This means that a sighted person cannot simply accept my company. Through no fault of his own, he has by walking with me deprived me of my independence.

Through no fault of my own, I have sacrificed my independence for the sake of his company. He then becomes responsible for me. He becomes like a car towing a caravan. It is his responsibility to make sure that the vehicle he is towing is still there, i.e. that I do not become detached from him at some crucial point of the route. He has to make sure that there is room, when passing between those two parked vehicles, not just for him, but for both of us. If he walks around the lamppost, but does not make sure that I walk round the lamppost, my collision with the lamppost will be his responsibility. All of this can be very unnerving for the inexperienced guide.

It is easy, in this situation, for the sighted person to assume that the dependency which he now finds himself committed to is my ordinary or typical state. He realizes that I am now depending on him for some warning of where the kerbs and the lampposts are, he finds it a little more difficult to imagine that, when I am alone, I can work these details out quite well for myself. He is thus always ready to rush up and give me his help, rather than merely to offer me his company, because his experience is always of my helplessness. Blindness creates a strange variation upon familiar human patterns of dependence and independence.

Stairs and Escalators   *7 July 1984*

Once he is on it, a stairway is one of the safest places for a blind person. You never find a chair left on a stairway, or a bucket or a brick. There is never a stair missing from a stairway, and all the stairs are the same height. There is almost always a handrail or at least a wall to touch. There may be some uncertainty about the top step and the bottom step, but with the white cane, that problem is simplified.

This puzzles most sighted people, who tend to assume that stairs will be dangerous for the blind. Sighted people know that they sometimes trip and fall on stairs, and they assume that, if a sighted person is likely to trip, a blind person is bound to.

It is very common when I am going up or down stairs for my sighted guide to count aloud the number of stairs, presumably for my benefit. Oddly enough, this is one of the few situations in which the additional knowledge is of little help or relevance. One can, of course, come upon a downward flight of stairs unexpectedly, and this would be as dangerous for a blind person as for a sighted one, and so the approach to a downward stair is an uncertain moment. The blind person needs to know two things: first, that he or she is approaching stairs, second, that the stairs go down. Most sighted guides disclose the first fact, very many, possibly a majority, forget about the second fact. The existence and the direction are essential; the number is immaterial. If I am descending a series of stairs interrupted by platforms, it is helpful to know when the last set of stairs has been completed, so that I can now set out confidently with my guide, not having to probe with my cane for the first stair of the next flight. Similarly, when approaching a circular stairway, it is helpful to know whether it will be curving clockwise or anticlockwise. A stairway can take an unexpected turn one way or the other, and it is easier on the outer edge of the curvature, where the steps are wider. Generally speaking, however, a stairway is a predictable structure. The same is true of lifts and of escalators.

What blind people find difficult are smooth, open spaces. It is just these areas which are assumed by many sighted people to be best for blind people, because there is no danger of tripping. From the blind point of view, however, a flat, open surface is not negotiable because there are no orientating signals. There is no structure. It is not predictable, because it may end at any moment, and there is no way of telling where you are, once you are on it. The problem for the blind person is not falling over, but knowing where he or she is. For this reason, it is easier to find my way around a campus which is marked out by steps, little hills and valleys, low walls and lots of changes in texture, because I can mark out my route with sections. The structure becomes a sequence when I am moving through it.

Let us take another example of an unpredictable structure. Sometimes my route over a forecourt is obstructed by cars parked at different angles from each other. The danger is not that I might walk into a car but that I will get lost. Blind people do sometimes walk into the edges of doors or into obstructions sticking out at head height, but it is unusual for a blind person to walk into a wall or a parked car. The white cane gives sufficient warning of the presence of such a large object. The problem is rather that having negotiated around three sides of the vehicle it is difficult to pick up one's route in exactly the same direction. If, with the next step, a second parked car is discovered, lying at a different angle, and then a third, it is almost impossible to align oneself with the original route. You have to try to maintain in your mind a map showing all these angles and set it against the original direction. This is what I call an unpredictable structure.

Learning from Cassettes   *8 July 1984*

Studying from cassettes means that the difference between the spoken word and the printed page is broken down. Reading a book has become like listening to a lecture. It is not quite the same, because by pressing the rewind button briefly I can get my lecturer to repeat again and again what she has been saying. Moreover, the recording means that there is no ambiguity about the actual words which were spoken, and I can listen to it again and again, from various points of view.

It remains true, however, that the task of summarizing a lecture or a speech as I am listening to it is very much the same whether the speaker is personally present on the platform or whether it is a recording. If you have the printed text in front of you as someone is speaking, you tend to follow the printed text, but if you have nothing but the speech, you have to concentrate entirely upon what is being said.

If I am getting any better at summarizing and evaluating immediate speech in the form of lectures and addresses, I am sure it is because of the practice I get in doing this very thing as I listen to books.

Becoming a Child   *9 July 1984*

I was walking along Navigation Street in the city centre. Someone offered me a packet of mints. 'Thank you,' I said brightly accepting the sweets with a cheerful smile.

'That's all right,' replied my benefactor. 'I had decided to give them to the next child I met anyway.'

At a formal dinner, the main course was chicken on the bone. I asked the person next to me to wave to the waitress, to ask the kitchen staff to take the chicken off the bone for me; this is the least embarrassing thing to do on these occasions. The guest next to me said that that would be quite unnecessary; she would cut up the chicken for me herself. This she did, very happily and skilfully, passing the plate back to me with the comment, 'I cut up a meal for a handicapped child only the other day.'

I was staying with a friend in an unfamiliar house, where there had been an overflow from the toilet during the night. The bathroom carpet was soaked with the overflow. My first knowledge of this was in the early morning, when I got up to go to the bathroom. My friend woke up immediately and called out, 'John, don't go into the bathroom. There's been an accident.'

I came back, and he explained the problem. As I sat thoughtfully on the edge of the bed, I said to him, 'Tell me, had you been lying there half awake all night, waiting for me to get up and go to the bathroom so you could intercept me in time? You didn't like to wake me up earlier to tell me? You knew it would be messy if I went in there without knowing?'

My very good, old friend gave me a laugh. 'Well,' he said, 'that's more or less right. I didn't stay awake. I went off to sleep, having set my head to wake up the moment I heard you get out of bed.' He added thoughtfully but with a chuckle, 'It's like having a child again.'

Travelling with my eleven-year-old daughter on British Rail, we could never work out whose ticket was whose. Her ticket, purchased on a Family Concession, had printed on it 'Flat Rate Fare'. Mine, purchased under a Disabled Person's Concession, had printed on it 'Child'.

I had a discussion the other day with Clive Inman, my medical friend, who has recently been recovering from a serious road accident, and is confined to a wheelchair. He tells me that when people see him in this wheelchair, they tend to speak to him in a gentle, slow and compassionate sort of voice. It is a kindly, condescending voice, the way some people speak to children. It is also the voice of uncertainty, people not knowing quite how to react in meeting an adult who has been 'cut down to size'.

A disabled adult man loses part of his manhood, part of his adulthood, and part of his humanity. I know Jesus told us we should repent and become as little children, but I don't want it in this way. I don't like having my adulthood wrenched from me like this.

The Power of Powerlessness   10 July 1984

While, on the one hand, it is so easy to be marginalized, it is also very easy to dominate. Sometimes blind people may not be aware of their dominance. One may not realize that one is the centre of a concern, that all around there is an elaborate fuss which involves getting out of one's way; preparations are being made for one, agreements are being reached about one, conversations are taking place in readiness for one's arrival. Sometimes, as a blind person I will realize that I am the centre of an attention which I do not want. I am an object of curiosity. All eyes are focused on me as I enter the room.

It is so hard to find an intermediate way, that is, somewhere between being ignored, and being the centre of attention. It is so hard to be a normal person when one is not a normal person. It is also hard to avoid the situation which arises when, because of one's very powerlessness, one does have a kind of power over people. The disabled person tends to render other people powerless. One flusters them, reduces them to confusion, covers them with uncertainty and embarrassment, makes them feel gauche and insensitive, awkward and intrusive, makes them realize that they do not know what to do, or that they are not handling this very well. The disabled person can inflict all of these feelings upon the normal.

To judge the right use of this power is an important part of learning to be a disabled person.

Feeling the Wind   *11 July 1984*

There is a certain point along my route which catches the wind. This morning, as I came up the steps from the underpass and around the corner, it hit me. It was a beautiful, warm, scented breeze, not hot like the Australian northerly, but full of a perfumed richness; a moving, fragrant wind. It was an unsettled wind, suggesting the break-up of rather a sultry day. I stood there for some time, allowing it to play over my face and through my clothes. I turned my head this way and that to catch its different currents. I leaned into it and away from it and breathed it in. It was delightful.

Can the wind mean as much to sighted people? It is invisible, so they gain nothing over blind people. Of course, blind people lose the sight of the world being blown along by the wind, the hurrying clouds and the trees swaying. On the other hand, the wind has a special beauty for blind people. For the sighted, to whom the world is mainly visual, an invisible phenomenon like the wind is only observed incidentally, it is one of many things which one notices in passing. It is mainly visual cues such as the sight of the washing blowing about on the line that give rise to the thought that it is a windy day. The wind itself, as felt by the body, is only one of the ways in which sighted people experience a windy day.

The blind person enters into the windiness of the day at first hand. For blind people, the wind does not have the enigmatic quality that it has for the sighted. There is a passage in the Fourth Gospel which says of the wind, 'You do not know where it goes or where it comes from'. I think that that is a sighted person's reaction, because sighted people are used to seeing where things go and where things come from. Sighted people work at long range. The sighted person tends to look at the pennants above the pavilion to see which way the wind is blowing.

Blind people are accustomed to not knowing where things come from and where they are going to. Things rush past: one is in the midst of a mêlée of action, one does not expect to see origins and destinations. The invisibility of the wind does not make it mysterious to blind people for whom there is no such thing as invisibility. The blind person experiences the impact of the wind upon his body and the sound of it in the trees. He knows perfectly well where it is coming from: it is coming from that direction, he is facing into it. The wind is coming from the direction I am facing when I face into it.

Sometimes a blind person experiences a wind which is all the more exciting because it is known at long range. I hear the distant tossing of trees across the park; it comes like a wave rolling across a beach. Now it breaks upon my body in a squall, a gust, like a fist. This is very exciting because of the anticipation, and the wonderful feeling of having the knowledge in your body of what is going on.

In what ways is the wind a symbol of the Holy Spirit for the blind?

Seeing with Your Fingers   *12 July 1984*

If I have to carry a cup of tea from this room into the next, I can do it. If you put a full glass into my other hand, then I cannot do it. Giving me a full glass in my second hand is like blindfolding me. A blind person with a full glass in each hand is equivalent to a sighted person blindfolded with a full glass in each hand. A blind person with a full glass in one hand only is roughly equivalent (I may be a bit slower and a bit more clumsy) to a sighted person with no blindfold and full glasses in each hand. It is the loss of the use of the second hand through having to hold a full glass which is equivalent to blindfolding. It might be objected that a blind person surely has the experience of being blindfolded, as it were, all the time. This, however, would be a mistake. As long as the blind person has one free hand, he or she sees with that hand. I do not experience not knowing where to go or where I am so long as I can guide myself with my free hand. I do not *feel* blind then, but with a full glass in each hand, it is almost impossible to avoid knocking against something and spilling a few drops. The only way to do it is to walk backwards, rubbing your back or elbows along the walls and so protecting the full glasses. To sighted people, this looks ridiculous.

It is difficult for a blind person to carry cups and plates on a tray from one room to another, or to carry a chair or anything which requires the use of both hands. If a blind person begins to forget what it was like to see, or if you want to explain to a blind person what it would be like for a sighted person to go blind, there would be no point in blindfolding the already blind person. What you do is put full tumblers of water into both of the blind person's hands and tell him to take them into the dining room. He will then bump into things, knock one or both glasses against corners and spill stuff, and will know exactly what it is like for a sighted person to be blindfolded.

Working the other way, a sighted person can always gain some understanding of what blindness is like by being blindfolded. This may be rather superficial unless one adds the additional blindfold, i.e. puts two glasses of water into the hands of the blindfolded sighted person, thus depriving her of guidance through the sense of touch. In other words, to obtain insight into the manoeuvrability problems of another mode of cognition it is not enough to delete the faculty most immediately affected (in our case, sight). One must allow the ramifications of this mode to be experienced by deleting a second sense (touch) showing how the nature of the second sense, and its usefulness within the mode as a whole, undergoes a change. Touch is not the same for the sighted person as it is for the blind person. Deleting sight but leaving touch untouched gives a false impression, because touch is affected when sight is deleted. In other words, blind people see with their fingers.

Training the Sighted   *13 July 1984*

Many of the people I mix with have never met a blind person. They have little idea of what to do or how to relate to me. I try to create situations in which sighted people will feel at home, but this is not always easy, and I often fail. I think that one reason for this failure is the fact that the relationship between the blind person and the sighted person is not often one of equality. Suppose I am standing, talking to people in a lounge bar. Suppose I have changed partners many times, using the technique described in 'Litmus Paper' above. Suppose now that I want to sit. I have several problems. Are there any unoccupied chairs in the room? How do I locate one?

I was talking to someone in this bar. It was during a residential conference. She pointed out that we had no drinks. I suggested that she should go to the bar and get drinks for both of us. I added that I would sit down and wait for her return. 'OK,' she said. 'Where would you like to sit?' I said, 'Why don't you take me to a chair, and put my hand on the back of it?' She took my hand and put it on the back of a chair, and off she went to the bar. I found that I was standing behind a lounge chair, but, on running my hand across the back of the chair, and down its sides in order to discover if the chair had arms or not, I found I was running my fingers across a woman's neck. There was someone sitting in the chair already. She got quite a surprise, for a strange man was feeling her neck and shoulders. There was general consternation, much laughter and apologies. Why, I wonder, didn't my first friend put my hand on the back of an empty chair? Had I somehow failed to make it clear that I wanted to sit down? Maybe my friend thought it was my intention merely to stand up with my hand on the back of a chair waiting for her.

When my friend came back from the bar with the drinks, she was apologetic, having seen the incident. We laughed and made our way towards some seats. I said, 'Let me put a finger under your left elbow if I may.' She would not let me do this. Instead, she stretched across with her own right hand, grasped my right hand firmly, pulled my forearm under her left arm, and closed her left arm tightly, continuing to hold my hand. This was someone who was determined not to make a second mistake. This time, there would be no ambiguity.

As we walked across the crowded lounge, I said to her brightly, 'You know, I have to train people the way they train guide dogs for the blind. I have a special technique for people to sit me down in an armchair. Wound you like me to train you in it?' Laughing, she agreed. 'OK,' I said. 'This is what we do. When we get to the chair, you take one of my hands, stretch it out, and place it on the back of the chair.'

When we got to the chair, she couldn't do this. Maybe the lounge chair was in an awkward position or something. I suggested that she should put her own hand on the back of the chair. She did this, by now thoroughly mystified. I simply ran my fingers along her arm and located the back of the chair. Immediately, I was orientated. I needed no further help. I knew exactly where the chair was, and I could now sit down any time I liked, with safety and dignity. My companion, however, refused to let go. 'Thank you,' I said cheerfully. 'That was very good. You can let go now and I will sit down.' She was determined to back me into the chair, holding both my elbows from the front. After a few more appeals I persuaded her to let go and I sat down. I contrast this with a similar incident which took place the following day. I was walking with another friend who said, 'Let's sit down.' In a swift, natural and unobtrusive movement she took my hand, placed it lightly on the back of a nearby armchair, and sat down herself on the adjacent chair without any further comment. I was so impressed by the speed and the gracious ease of this gesture, that I asked her if she was used to working with blind people. 'I never met a blind person in my life before,' she said, 'but I get a fast read-out.' This person, as I got to know her, proved to be someone of exceptional sensitivity and insight.

Yes, I begin to think that I really do have a sort of a litmus test. What degree of freedom will this new person be prepared to allow me? Will this sighted person find ways of letting me preserve as much independence and dignity as possible? Will this person want to possess me, to control me, to make me feel even more handicapped by refusing to admit that I can do the slightest thing for myself? For my part, how can I make it easier for sighted people? My policy of giving cheerful, simple directions will work with some, but not with others.

Does He Take Sugar? 16 July 1984

At church, one of the vergers approached Marilyn as she was standing with me, and said to her, 'Marilyn, is it John's wish to go forward to the Communion Rail?' Marilyn made no reply, so I turned towards him and said with a smile, 'Yes, thank you very much, I will be going forward.' There was a slight sound of surprise, and I gathered that the kindly man was somewhat flustered because I had overheard what he had said. I assured him that I would be quite all right, and would go up accompanied by Marilyn as I normally did. I thanked him for his concern. I think that he was assuming I was deaf. Why not tap me on the elbow, and ask me whether I intended to go forward, and whether I would need any assistance? I would appreciate this thoughtful gesture. To speak *about* me, in the third person, to someone else, is another matter.

This situation often seems to arise when I am getting in a car with a group of other people. 'Will you put John in the back with you?' 'No, I'll put him in the front with you.' 'All right, you put him in then.' At this point I interjected, crying out with an exceedingly loud voice, 'John is not *put* anywhere, thank you very much. John is asked if he has any preferences about where he sits.' At this, all my friends laughed uproariously and were covered with apologies and confusions. On a similar occasion recently I shouted out, 'Hey, you guys, don't you talk about me as if I'm not here.' This, again, brought shouts of laughter and a mixture of apologies, agreements and congratulations.

It is, of course, very embarrassing for intelligent and sensitive people when they are caught out like this, in using the 'does he take sugar?' approach to a disabled person. These people are all sensitive, and well aware of the humiliation which this approach implies. So the question arises, why do they do it?

It is so easy to marginalize a blind person, indeed, in certain situations it is almost impossible not to.

Visiting Melbourne 29 July 1984

I had been nervous about several aspects of this visit. I had been afraid of a renewed sense of loss through being in a place which has so many visual memories for me. Flinders Street Station and Princes Bridge, St Paul's Cathedral, and the famous view of the city seen over the River Yarra from the Botanical Gardens, these are all sights which are deeply etched upon my mind. I have always loved the view along Collins Street towards the Victorian parliament buildings, and the vistas along St Kilda Road, with the Shrine of Remembrance standing out so prominently among the lawns and trees.

In the case of Birmingham, I have had time to adjust to the gradual disappearance of well-loved buildings, and to revise my memories bit by bit as people tell me about demolitions here and reconstructions there. To be suddenly plunged back as a blind person into a world so full of remembered visions made me feel most unhappy. I felt particularly dismayed by the thought that I would not be able to enjoy the coastline. I had always loved Port Philip Bay with its lapping waves and myriads of yachts, but my greatest excitement had always been the south-western Victorian coast. Here the Great Ocean Road, cut out of the cliff, takes you through spectacular scenery, down to the Port Campbell area, where the massive waves have eroded strange shapes in the cliffs, and the wildness and majesty of the scenery had always held a strong fascination for me. Although I had never been a great lover of the outdoor life as such, and could claim almost no real experience of bush walking, I had always been moved by the endless ridges of blue-grey hills and the gaunt beauty of the rocky outcrops of granite. The Grampian Mountains had been a favourite holiday spot for us children, since my mother had been brought up as a child in the nearby town of Stawell. When I was there in the spring of 1980, many of the best-remembered places were already inaccessible to me because of my poor vision and the rocky, uneven ground. Wonderland, the Grand Canyon, the Nerve Test, the Whale, the Fallen Giant and the Elephant's Hide were already fading. Now they would be entirely gone.

I was most anxious about the people I was to meet. I knew that it would undoubtedly cause pain to people I knew and loved so much when they met me as a blind person. I felt worried and rather frightened at the thought that I would have to reconstitute my knowledge of them on the basis of sound and touch, just as I was doing with people I was not meeting for the first time in England. All of my visual memories of those loved faces were now at best an irrelevance and at worst an actual obstruction to my entering into a real and contemporary relationship with them.

I also felt disturbed at the thought of being deprived of my routine for so many weeks. I would have to learn my way round so many new houses and buildings, make myself familiar with new household utensils, and learn the names of so many new people. I felt afraid that in this situation I would be even more thoroughly marginalized, even more completely passive than I always am these days.

I have to admit that all of these fears were fulfilled. After three or four days I developed persistent asthma which has not really lifted after ten or twelve days. I have been aware of quite a severe sense of suffering, even of anguish. One of the strands of this is realizing that people who love me are trying to communicate with me. They are having to get used to me again, like this. My mother sat close beside me at the nature reservation, while the children fed a tiny wallaby with a bottle of milk. She stroked my hand lightly, saying, 'I have to touch you because I feel that's the only way I can get close to you now.' I longed for a more immediate recognition of loved ones than the rather slow, day-by-day building up of impressions, histories and voices which blindness seems to require.

In the presence of those from whom I have been absent for so long, I want something more than this. I want to be in the immediate presence, to have the same person again. I want to be greeted by the person I love in his or her remembered form. Not being able to experience this is a cause not only of frustration but of grief.

The loss of the sights of the city, the sea and the countryside, I can endure. There is, however, a problem of sharing. It is so difficult to remain always interested and enthusiastic when people are pointing things out and reminding me of the lovely view which one can see from this spot. I sense their own perplexity at how they can help me to share their own enjoyment, how to show things off, how to be proud about the recent developments, how to draw me into this world which they love so much.

I still have difficulty in renouncing my role as father, as the convivial one who always makes others feel at home. How can I any longer count upon being reliable as good company? How can I any longer take the initiative in anecdotes and witticisms? What about my role as leader and guide to my own children? I am sharply conscious of the difficulty of showing the place off to them. As we travel around, I want to say, 'Look! That is where we did so-and-so. There is the place where it happened. Down that street I once lived. There! You can just catch a glimpse of my old school.' I cannot even point out the strange animals to the children unless I get a description first of what they look like.

I have been driving myself on with the expectation that I would and should be able to do all these things. During the first ten or twelve days

I was fighting to bring my emotions under control, and felt almost continually on the edge of exhaustion and panic. The defences which I have built up were being threatened.

In the middle of all this, I had a strangely impressive dream. I was going to Cambridge to register for a Master of Theology degree. I was to enrol at Gonville and Caius College. Suddenly I was myself required to sit the final paper, with all the other candidates who had, however, been able to pursue the course the whole year. I was struggling with the examination questions, knowing that I was at a considerable disadvantage. After the examination, I was presented with a financial statement of what the year would cost me, if I was successfully enrolled. This was given to me by the Reverend Jack Newport (who had actually been my tutor when I was at Cambridge from 1959 to 1962). The bill amounted to £2,600 and with a shock I realized that I had not yet made any applications to trusts for grants. I would have to take immediate steps to make it clear to the college authorities that the work I had done on the examination paper should not be considered in the same light as the papers done by the other candidates, because there had been a terrible misunderstanding. I should not even have been taking that examination. The rest of the dream consisted in wandering around this beautifully furnished old college, with its lovely displays of antiques, its thronging students everywhere, its strange and interesting doors with the impressive names of members of staff with whom one had to make appointments.

The thing that stuck in my mind was that I was being judged in a context full of associations of a beautiful past which was, however, misunderstanding me, and to which I could probably not now gain access. I am blaming myself for being blind, accusing myself of being on the margin, critical of myself for not doing more for my parents, my wife and my children. I blame myself that I cannot give them a better life, that I cannot make it good for them to be here, in this wonderful country.

One thing which I did not feel, compared with my trip here more than four years ago, was the sense of resentment against the sighted world. I did not feel as if I wanted to withdraw from the world of sighted people and lose myself in the less demanding and more comfortable world of blind people who would understand me.

I have been helped a lot through the present crisis by Marilyn who keeps telling me that I must not put myself under such demands, that I must not have such expectations. I have also been comforted by applying to myself the words from the famous sermon by Paul Tillich, 'You are accepted'. I am accepted in my blindness. I am accepted as a blind person.

I have been helped by two other things. First, the primary school at which my elder sister teaches has made an office available for my use. She picks me up in her car every morning on her way to school, and I have my tape recorders in the office there. I work there all the school day, joining the staff for the tea breaks and at lunchtime. After school, I return with my sister and spend the rest of the late afternoon and evening with the family and relatives. This has established a pattern which is giving me a sense of familiarity. Secondly, I have discovered that I can control the attacks of asthma by breathing. I must have seen dozens of doctors over the years about asthma, but none has ever told me that I could reduce my panic and thus diminish the actual attack by a simple technique of breathing. I have discovered it over the past two or three days. By breathing from the stomach, I can stop wheezing. After a dozen or twenty breaths the sense of panic passes, and breathing becomes easier. Instead of being frightened by the thought that I could be dead in three or four minutes, I now know that I am already up to the seventh or eight breath, and within another ten or twelve the worst will be over. It works, it is like fighting an enemy.

Places   *30 July 1984*

Maybe my earlier view that one place is like another was exaggerated. Yesterday the whole family went to a place called Fairy Park, about twenty miles inland from Geelong. This is a granite outcrop, worn into huge boulders intersected with gulleys and ravines, laid out as a barbecue area with a winding trail through the boulders, into which are set scenes of fairy-tales. These animated models are behind glass-like shop windows. The children ran from one to the next with great excitement, pressing the buttons which set the displays in motion, turning on the music and the story.

I came away with quite a vivid impression of this place. I did not feel remote and abstract, perhaps because I was able to take an active part, in lifting the children up to see better, or so they could press the buttons, and because the nursery rhymes and fairy-tales were familiar, so there was plenty to talk about. Having direct acoustic access to the displays was important. I knew what was going on, because of the commentary. I was in demand from the children to answer questions, and to hold buttons pressed down and so on. There was also the walking itself, up and down little slopes, passing through the gaps between boulders, a series of little ravines, feeling the rough stone on either side, going into caves or other covered areas and feeling the difference in the echoes, the

105

changes in temperature as we moved from an exposed place where the breeze was quite cool into a secluded place where the air was still warm and we could feel the sunlight. We came to the highest point, a look-out place, and I could feel the handrail. I could sense the vast, open space, the drop at my feet. The movement of air was so different, and whereas before I could hear the echoing footsteps of the running children, now it was the cries of the wheeling gulls, the noise coming from the distant brick kiln down in the valley, the patterns of the roads beneath me traced out by the passing traffic and the excited comments of the sighted people gathered along the rail next to me. Finally, we came back to the picnic area, where there was the fascinating feel of the rough-hewn wooden benches and the different kinds of tessellated pavements linking the various facilities. The fact that we had gone around the entire area and come back helped me to realize the dimensions of the place and made me feel it was distinctive.

Growing Old Together   *31 July 1984*

To grow old together is to experience the passage of time so intimately that the ageing process is shared. There are, however, various kinds and degrees of intimacy. Let us suppose that you and I are walking together in the hills. We exchange conversation; I see the expressions on your face – your admiration of the view, your amusement as a squirrel runs across our path. Your inner life is available to me not only in your face but in your posture, in the whole of your bodily movements. We are face to face with each other, in mutual awareness.

There is a second situation in which our awareness is no longer mutual, although we are still together. You are reading a book and I am watching you. You do not know I am watching you. Perhaps you even drop off to sleep, and I continue to observe you. Perhaps I am playing chess with my friend while you are watching TV and also observing us from the corner of your eye. We, however, are absorbed in the game.

There is still a third situation in which rather than being conscious of each other, or one conscious of the other, we are both sharing an experience which absorbs us. If you and I are out driving and a huge truck careers towards us from the other side of the motorway, we are not conscious of each other's reactions. All attention is focused upon the danger and on the split-second actions being taken to avoid the collision. Only afterwards do we turn to one another and say 'What went through your mind when you saw that truck coming?' Similarly, you and I are watching a bird in flight. We are doing this together and I am dimly conscious of the movements of your head as you too follow the diving bird. If my attention is no longer on the bird but on you, we revert to the second situation, and if we both forget about the bird and turn towards each other, we revert to the first situation, that of being face to face. But as long as we are both concentrating on the flight of the bird, we are mutually experiencing life; we are together in the flow of time; the event passes over both of us simultaneously; we are together, and growing older together. The passage of time, the experience of the moments is shared by both of us as we plunge into them. It is this participation in the flow of experience which is the essence of what Alfred Schutz calls in his writings 'growing older together'.

There is no doubt that blindness affects all three of these basic situations. We must distinguish between blind people relating to each other and the sighted relating to the blind. The main point about the latter situation is its lack of reciprocity. To you, my sighted friend, I am present as an object in your visual field along with the other people we are with and the furniture and other things in the room. You speak to me and to our sighted friends. You may adapt your behaviour towards me; nevertheless, you see all of us. Blindness, however, is a subjective state. There is no longer a field of vision, a pictorial world within which people and things are placed. The blind person must make a mental note of who is at the meeting, and a conscious effort of memory all the time. The sighted people at the meeting do not have to make any such conscious effort of memory – all alike, blind and sighted, are obviously there.

A common deterioration of mutuality takes place when a blind and a sighted person believe, or one of them believes that they are in a face-to-face situation but in fact you, the sighted one, are looking out of the window. I lean forward expectantly waiting for your next remark but you are reading a letter. You are no longer paying attention to me, but I do not know that. Similarly, you gaze at me, wondering if I am listening. Perhaps I have dropped off to sleep. Perhaps I am thinking. We seem to share the same space and time but the fact that I cannot read your emotions and experiences in your face and in the movement of your body means that the sharing is no longer so intimate. The data of togetherness have become meagre.

If we turn to the third of these situations, the mutual sharing of an experience, we can see how blindness impoverishes this. The mere fact that blind and sighted people cannot watch things together, obvious though this is, deprives them of a major field of togetherness. Indeed, we can listen together, but how can we have mutual experience of our common listening? We sit in seats next to each other, listening to the orchestra. But how can I tell if you are engrossed in the music or not? If I were sighted, I would see the tapping of your foot, the lines of concentration on your brow and we would exchange a glance or a smile when the music rose to a climax. I would enjoy your amusement when the conductor dropped the baton.

Can merely holding hands be an effective substitute? Touch, of course, is reciprocal but unless there is a returning pressure one does not know if there is real reciprocity or not. I may hold your hand but you may be asleep. You give a little squeeze, but what does it mean? Does not the knowledge 'we are listening together and having similar emotions' depend upon the visual availability of each to the other?

The mere fact that I find myself wondering how you are reacting means that our relationship has become an object of conscious thought and thus the immediacy of unselfconscious participation in an event is already lost. It is thus more difficult to establish that blind and sighted people really share the same social and emotional time and space.

Another aspect of the mutuality which is to some extent impoverished lies in the way in which the emotional life of one person is mirrored by and in another. As a sighted friend, I see the dawn of anxiety on your face perhaps before you yourself have realized it. Before the thought that you are anxious has formed in your own mind, I know you are anxious. There is thus an anticipation, a sort of witness beforehand, which greatly enriches the mutuality of the experiences of sighted friends.

The failure of the blind and the sighted to live in the same process of time becomes clearer if we realize that this mirroring, this mutual witnessing, is diminished. As a blind person, I can only become aware of your anxiety if you speak. It is true that I may immediately detect anxiety in your voice which you did not know was there, but if you make no sound at all, I am separated from you. It is true that the moment I touch your hand, I may sense your tension, your anxiety. But if we are out of reach, that too is lost. My awareness of your inner emotional state thus tends to lag behind your own awareness of it, rather than being the witness and mirror of it. You must recognize your own emotions; only occasionally can you discover your emotions reflected beforehand from me.

Submarine   *13 August 1984*

Last Friday I had a very impressive dream. It was set entirely in the depths of the ocean. Nothing was shown above the surface at all. It was a bit like scenes from the film *Ice Station Zebra*, I think it was called, about a nuclear submarine going under the ice cap, except that in the dream there was no ice cap; it was just deep under the ocean, very murky. The dream was divided between scenes of the outside of the submarine and those of the inside. This huge hulk, rather like a gigantic, elongated, flying saucer equipped with jet engines, was travelling through the depths of the ocean. It was not long and thin, as a submarine might be, but bulky and round. The view of the inside of the submarine showed the crew trying to interpret their instruments. They did not know whether the craft was travelling forwards or backwards. I myself was not in the dream; I was viewing all this, as if at the cinema. The crew were intently watching the screens upon which the water outside the submarine was displayed. They were covered with disappearing, fluctuating, luminous traces, rather like the ones I now see in my right eye. There was a discussion about whether these traces were approaching the vessel or leaving it. Finally, there was a picture, from the outside, of the submarine touching the bottom of the sea. A very perilous situation had been reached. The main impression left by the dream was of a huge, lumbering weight, of vast power advancing steadily, but with those in charge not knowing which way it was going.

There was no trace of blindness in this dream. It was in beautiful, impressive colour. There were the deep blues and greens of the ocean, the lights of the moving submarine, its grey and white hulk, the luminous trails that it left behind as it moved.

It is strange how much I have come to depend upon dreams for entertainment. I am engrossed in dreams like this, rather as I might have been fascinated by watching an epic film. The outside world seldom comes home to me with such vividness.

Although the dream was powerful, and portrayed a situation of great peril, it also conveyed to my waking mind a sort of friendliness, as if the depths are aware of my problem, and are trying to help me, to describe things for me. The submarine is blind, and sees as I do. But the ocean is also blind, and the submarine moves through it, trying to find direction and contact. Now I am the ocean; now I am the submarine. I am also the submarine and the ocean at the same time. The dream is me and yet it is greater than me.

I arrived in Melbourne with the family about a month ago. This is the long-awaited visit to my relatives, and the long-feared attempt to get to know my parents again as a blind person. My parents have been marvellous, most understanding and matter of fact. I still find the experience particularly difficult and distressing, to be cut off in this way from the people one loves most, to have to begin again, as it were, without the faces of one's own mother and father.

Melbourne is where my childhood lies. Here, I always have a strange experience of encounter with that past. I left Australia for study in England at the age of twenty-four. This is the fourth time I have been back. Visiting my parents always makes me aware of the connection between my faith in God and my relationship with them. I have no doubt that my lifelong love affair with God is, at least partly, an expression of my lifelong attempt to know and love my father, and to be known and loved by him.

6

Round the Bend

Autumn 1984

Lecturing without Notes   *19 August 1984*

I have now spent about four years grappling with the problem of how to speak in public without notes. As a sighted lecturer, I never had to read from a text, except when trying to present a particularly closely argued section. Usually all I needed was a list of headings, divided into sections with subheadings. Of course, if I was giving the sort of lecture which involved a lot of historical facts or statistics, then I would refer to a printed text.

After loss of sight, I tried various ways of dealing with this problem. I experimented in making a summary on micro-cassette which I would use as a prompt. The problem was, that if I happened not to need the reminder until later in the lecture, I would have to run the cassette through all the material until arriving at the point, and this would take a few seconds. Locating the exact point was very difficult, and it was an embarrassing disclosure to an audience that one had lost the way.

Sometimes I would record a brief summary of what I proposed to say, divided into sections. I would actually play this short summary to my audience, and would simply talk around it. This was only a partial success. Sometimes my listeners found it difficult to hear what was coming out of the tape recorder and I would have to repeat it, which was time-wasting. It was also inflexible, in that it committed me to an invariable sequence and to a great deal of laborious preparation, and these factors impaired my informal style and my capacity to respond to the needs of the moment.

I tried dictating to myself by making a recording of the whole speech, or a summary, and using an earplug. For a while I actually tried to listen and speak at the same time, but after one or two disastrous experiences I gave this up. I tried using braille headings. This not only involved laborious preparation, but my braille was just not good enough. I could not scan quickly enough to get myself out of the difficulty which arose when I forgot what to say next.

In the end, I developed the habit of making a précis on cassette and of listening and re-listening to this right up to the moment when I had to deliver the lecture. I would take the tape recorder to the lecture, since it gave me a sense of security, although I seldom needed to refer to it.

During a teachers' course in Canterbury in the spring of 1982, I was sitting in my room feverishly listening to this summary when I was called to the lecture theatre by an old friend. When she realized what I was doing, she told me off. 'Just forget all that rubbish,' she said. 'You won't forget it. Just come and talk to us.' I did, and it was a great success.

I now seem to have developed a way of scanning ahead in my mind, to work out what I am going to say. Everybody does this in ordinary speech, otherwise we couldn't complete a sentence. Somehow or other, and without effort, I have developed a longer perspective, and now when I am speaking I can see paragraphs coming up from the recesses of my mind. It is a bit like reading them off a scanner. While I am speaking, another part of my mind is sorting out into paragraphs what I am going to be saying in the next few minutes, and a yet more remote part is selecting alternative lines of argument from a sort of bank of material. This seems to give my lecturing style a greater sense of order than I had before, and people seem to be able to follow me more easily.

I can often cross-reference what I have said, that is, I can remind my audience of a point I made under subheading 2(a) fifteen minutes ago. People find this surprising, but it is not surprising. If I did not have the material in sections like that I would not be able to maintain the argument at all. That particular little habit has come, I think, from hearing students' essays read to me. Often one of my readers will be slightly surprised when I say, 'Go back to what was said on page 3 under section 4(f).' I have not put any particular effort into learning how to do this; it is just that it is so inconvenient if you have to have the whole essay read again. You tend to make unconscious mental notes of the structure so that you can go back to it again if necessary. Of course, often it doesn't work, either because I am not concentrating sufficiently or because the structure in what is being read to me is too vague. It is, however, a kind of mental skill which studying from cassettes has, I suppose, forced upon me.

A sighted author tends to paragraph his or her work retrospectively. You see the stuff unrolling on the typewriter or screen, and you think that it is about time you started a new paragraph. A person listening to books on cassettes, where the actual paragraphs in the printed page are not normally indicated, does his or her own paragraphing, and when composing tends to project this into the future of the composition. I think that this also helps me to organize my material in advance when I am speaking in public. A sighted lecturer reading from a typescript concentrates mainly upon what she has said, that is, the paragraphs slip away behind her as she 'swims' forward through her speech. As a blind speaker I have to concentrate entirely upon what I am about to say, or what I will be saying fifteen minutes from now, because otherwise I will lose direction. It is rather fallible, but it does seem to be turning into a method which will often work.

Seeing Lizzie   *21 August 1984*

Last night I had a vivid dream in colour. I dreamt that I had got out of bed, and was kneeling or sitting beside the bed, perhaps looking for my slippers or something. This little toddler came padding into the room. I could see her quite clearly in the dim light. In the dream, I knew that I had been blind, and that this was the first time I had been able to see her. I stared at her, full of wonder, taking in every detail of her face as she stood there wreathed in smiles, stretching out her hands to me. It was like a revelation. I thought, 'So this is her. This is the smile they all talk about. These are those luminous, brown eyes.' I had a wonderful sense of a renewal of contact, as I felt that she was amazed as she realized, in some way, that there was something different about me, that I was responding to her in a new sort of way. We stood there in complete silence, or, at least, I sat there and she stood beside me. We gazed at one another in this moment of mutual delight. Then the dream faded.

Was this a little dream or a big dream? Was it mere wish-fulfilment or was this an example of what Jung calls the archetype of the divine child, a kind of dream which he reports from his patients when a new self was at the point of birth. The child who visited me in the night was radiant with grace.

'Can't You See Colours?'   *21 August 1984*

This morning as I was drying him after his bath, Thomas asked me which towel I had used to dry Lizzie. I replied that I did not know, and he asked me, 'Was it the white one?' Again, I said that I did not know, and he asked, 'Would Mummy know?'

When I said 'Yes', he asked why Mummy would know.

'Because Mummy can see colours.'

'Can't you see colours?'

'No.'

'Why can't you see colours?'

'Because I can't see anything. I'm blind.'

'Oh.'

The concept of being unable to see has so many fragments. The child does not put these together into one global idea, any more than the adult does. Many adults do not immediately grasp the fact that it is no use saying to a blind person that something is over there. The words 'here' and 'there' have to be used in a different way with blind people. We may say that such an adult has not realized the linguistic implication of blindness. The child may not realize the colour implication of blindness. An adult might be surprised at the thought that a child would not realize that a blind person could not see colours, but then a blind person might be surprised that a sighted person did not realize the verbal implication of blindness.

This was the first discussion I have had with Thomas about colour, although about a week ago an incident occurred which brought home to him the mobility problems of the blind. It took a long time for me to learn the layout of our Melbourne home. As I was getting out of the car, I tried to go towards the front door of the house alone. I turned along the left-hand side of the house instead of the right and one of the other adults called me back. 'This way, John.' Laughing, Thomas said, 'He was going the wrong way. He would have gone towards the gate.' He kept repeating this, surprised and amused, as we walked along the path. I am not sure if he connected my mistake with blindness, or whether he merely thought I had done something funny.

Mr Treloar   11 September 1984

While I was in Melbourne I seized the opportunity to ask my mother about the origin of her Christian faith. I received my own faith by way of my parents, and that faith cannot be traced back very far on my father's side. His own father was a Unitarian but my father, Jack Hull, after emigrating to Australia as a lad during the First World War, not only drifted out of all association with church life, but in his middle twenties became quite an active atheist. The immediate human influence in his later conversion was provided by the committed Christian woman (whom he later married) who happened to be running the one-teacher school in the settlement where my father was the machine operator in the sawmill. This was in the Dandenong ranges, about thirty or forty miles north-east of Melbourne.

I had never been quite clear about the source of my mother's own faith. I knew that she had been brought up in a country town in north-western Victoria, not far from the Grampian mountains. It was called Stawell, and was famous mainly for its foot-race, the Stawell Gift. I had revisited Stawell with my mother and father, together with Marilyn and Imogen, in April of 1980. She had pointed out to me the Congregational church which she used to attend as a child. Her father, Alf Huttley, had died while I myself was but a child, and I cannot even remember him. He was a man of some enterprise, and started the first garage in Stawell. The cars were imported by sea from England. He used to go down to Melbourne and drive them back. Alf and his wife Alice used to attend the Congregational church in Stawell, and Alf was the conductor of the choir. From him my mother got her love of music. As a teenager, she used to be one of the pianists with the Stawell Choral Society, and taught me early in life to love such works as Handel's *Messiah* and Stainer's *Crucifixion*. My mother never spoke of her own parents, however, as being anything other than fairly conventional church people. I do not think that she could have received her own lively and independent faith from them.

I have now learnt that during the final year of her secondary school education, my mother transferred from Stawell High School to Melbourne High School, which was in those days co-educational. It is odd that I myself moved from Bendigo High School to the second year of the sixth form in Melbourne High School, many years later, at a time when my father took up his first appointment in the Victorian capital.

When she had finished this year at Melbourne High School, my mother spent a year as a trainee teacher in a primary school in Caulfield, another suburb of Melbourne, and the same area where I myself happened to begin my teaching career.

During these two years in Melbourne my mother lodged with the Treloar family. I had met Mildred Treloar on a number of occasions, knowing her as a lifelong friend of my mother. She spent most of her working life as an Evangelical Protestant missionary in India, and has, in fact, only recently died. I had always had the impression that Mildred, who was a robust personality, had had a deep influence upon my mother's own outlook, but I had never realized the circumstances under which they first met. It seems that while my mother was staying in Melbourne during those two years she began to go to a weekly Bible class with Mildred, who was about her own age. For the first time in her life, she began to read the Bible seriously, and with interest and a sense of responsibility. Over a period of several months, her personal dedication was renewed and deepened, as the pages of the Bible became more alive to her. It is to this period of her life that she looks back for the human origin of her Christian faith.

Now, where did Mildred Treloar find her faith? She got it from her father. He had wanted to enter the ministry of one of the Protestant churches, I am not sure if it was the Methodist or the Congregational, but had not been permitted to proceed because he lost his sight. The curious thing is that I myself at the age of nineteen, having conceived a desire to enter the ministry of the Methodist church, was enormously distressed to find that the church authorities were reluctant to accept me because of the poor state of my own sight, and the threat of blindness which was already hanging over me. I can distinctly remember one of the older, responsible ministers with whom I had an interview pointing out to me that if I should lose my sight I would become a burden upon the church, and they would then have to maintain me out of the retirement funds. I was surprised and a little shocked by this interview, and am now intrigued by the thought that a somewhat similar incident had occurred in the life of the young man who was to become the father of Mildred Treloar. My mother tells me that she has very vivid memories of herself as a girl of eighteen reading to old Mr Treloar, taking it in turns with Mildred. She describes him as a radiant Christian and still remembers quite clearly a sermon which he preached, late in his life, about the Christian hope of heaven. She says that as he spoke of the next world, his face was transformed with hope and joy. That must have been round about the year 1920.

It is interesting to think that that old, blind preacher should have been able to send his faith forward over an interval of more than sixty years, where it now illumines the life of another blind man. It is curious that he should have passed his faith to his daughter, who passed it on to her country friend, who passed it on to the atheist saw-mill operator, who with her, passed it on to their son, who was to lose his own sight and so, perhaps, begin the whole cycle again. I should like to know where old Mr Treloar got his faith from, but my mother did not know, or could not remember. I suppose it does not really matter. That old, blind man is my witness.

'Open Your Eyes. I Can't Hear You' *14 September 1984*

Partially deaf people are reported to hear better in a lighted room than in the darkness. Improved hearing takes place even when a candle is lit. If a note is struck on a piano in a totally dark room, while the light is turned on and off, the sound will appear to come and go. This effect does not appear if the eyes are closed or covered. Spectacles have been known to improve people's hearing.

This is called synesthesia, the working together of the senses. It is particularly noticeable in people under the influence of hallucinogenic drugs, who report seeing brightly coloured lights when loud, high-pitched notes are struck. It is also said to be more vivid in children than in normal adults, and children are sometimes heard to exclaim, 'Open your eyes! I can't hear you.'

This seems to contradict the widespread belief that when you go blind, your hearing improves. The fact would seem to be that without the support of sight, perception of sound actually deteriorates. This would also explain why so frequently I feel that I am not being listened to. It is not just a social difficulty in knowing when to intervene and in knowing when I have people's attention. Sighted people actually find it more difficult to hear what I say, because they cannot catch my eyes. Eye contact improves audibility, but the blind tend to become inaudible.

The Underground *19 September 1984*

Last Friday I really enjoyed travelling on the London Underground. The surfaces are smoother to walk on than the street-level footpaths. I learned a better way of getting on and off the escalators, which pleased me, and I found the winds in the tunnels rather interesting. As the trains come in and out, currents of air are pushed along the platforms, up the stairways and along the tunnels. These are full of the fragrance of newspaper, metals and oils, together with traces of cigar smoke, food and people's clothes.

Most interesting was the train itself. Between stations, there is nothing to be seen through the windows, so I did not feel frustrated about missing the view. I found I could easily distinguish the metallic click of the wheels on the rails, the electronic hum of the engines as the train gathered power, the swish of the automatic doors opening and closing, and the rushing noise of the air in the tunnel itself. The sound of the wind when you are approaching a platform is quite different from when you are leaving it. As well as all this, there are the human noises, the conversation in the compartment, the rustle of clothes and the footsteps as people get in and out, and the whole background noise of the station which comes flooding into the compartment each time the doors are opened. The whole panorama is repeated every two or three minutes, this being the time it takes to travel from one station to the next. There is the rapid acceleration, faster and faster until we reach our maximum speed. The brakes are applied and the deceleration commences. We roar into a new station, stop with a jerk, and the whole process begins again. Moreover, the sounds entirely envelop me. I am in the middle of them.

Presence   *20 September 1984*

I have realized that the intensity of my feeling of blindness is in proportion to my presence with people whose lives I long to share. I am, for example, not particularly conscious of being blind when I am at work. Most of what I do in the University is done on my terms. People have to fit in with my diary, come to my room, get used to my things, and my way of working. Our sharing is more a sharing of ideas than of our lives as such.

With family, it is otherwise. Over this weekend, I have become sharply aware of how much sighted children live in a visual world. Their play, their humour, their dressing-up and their tumbling around, everything is in the context of sight. It is by way of contrast with this that I developed a sense that I am not in the presence of these sighted children.

I am, of course, an object in their visual field, but the world of common experience, the world which we know together, the world before which we stand in a sort of mutuality of presence, that is so fragmented by blindness.

Rainfall and the Blind Body   *21 September 1984*

At five o'clock this morning I woke up to the sound of rain. I went into my study and pressed my forehead against the window pane. The house was completely still, and the streets outside seemed to be deserted. I stood there motionless, hardly breathing, concentrating everything upon the sound of the rain.

First, I noticed differences of place. Some sounds come from the left of the window, some from the right, and I can trace these as far as the corner of the house and around it. Now I pay attention to the higher sounds, as the rain splatters on the wall above the window and on the

118

roof of the house itself. Below me, the rain falls on to a fence, the shrubbery and on to the ground itself.

Next, there are differences of speed. There is a slow, steady drip, drip, drip, and a more rapid cascade, against the background of the pitter-patter of the individual drops on the window pane. These vary in speed as the rainstorm itself ebbs and flows, and some patterns of sounds overtake others, a bit like the music of Steve Reich.

I notice now that there are differences in intensity. Here a surface is meeting the full force of the rain but here is a sheltered place. Over there is a heavy splashing, not the sound of rain at all, but of collected water overflowing from a blocked pipe or something like that.

Differences of pitch emerge. There is the high-pitched drumming staccato as the drops fall on metal, the deeper, duller impact on brick or concrete, and I notice that the note being struck differs slightly even from one window pane to another. There are differences in the speed with which the water is travelling, it swishes, gurgles, pelts along in a fury, comes and goes. There are differences in the volume. On the window pane, it is very loud. The panes of glass vibrate on my forehead. The sounds diminish, layer upon layer, receding into the faint distance as the rain falls on nearby trees. I wonder how far away I can hear it falling. Can I make it out on the houses over the road? I can certainly hear it on the house next door.

This built up into a complex pattern. The more intensely I listened, the more I found I could discriminate, building block upon block of sound, noticing regularities and irregularities, filling dimension upon dimension. Complete silence was necessary. Even the slight sound of my breathing was enough to obscure some of the faintest details. It reminded me of the noise of the London Underground, which was similarly patterned into many textures, layers and shapes, so many positions and levels.

Is it true that the blind live in their bodies rather than in the world? I am aware of my body just as I am aware of the rain. My body is similarly made up of many patterns, many different regularities and irregularities, extended in space from down there to up here. These dimensions and details reveal themselves more and more as I concentrate my attention upon them. Nothing corresponds visually to this realization. Instead of having an image of my body, as being in what we call the 'human form', I apprehend it now as these arrangements of sensitivities, a conscious space comparable to the patterns of the falling rain. The patterns of water envelop me in myriads of spots of awareness, and my own body is presented to me in the same way. There is a central area, of which I am

119

barely conscious, and which seems to come and go. At the extremities, sensations fade into unconsciousness. My body and the rain intermingle, and become one audio-tactile, three-dimensional universe, within which and throughout the whole of which lies my awareness. This is in sharp contrast to the single-track line of consecutive speech which makes up my thoughts. This line of thought expressed in speech is not extended in space at all, but comes towards me like carriages in a goods train, one after the other, coming out of the darkness, passing under the floodlight of knowledge, and receding into memory. That line of consecutive thoughts is situated within the three-dimensional reality of the patterns of consciousness made up by the rain and my body, a bit like the axis of a spinning-top. It could be otherwise, however. If the rain were to stop, and I remain motionless here, there would be silence. My awareness of the world would again shrink to the extremities of my skin. If I were paralysed from the neck down, the area would again be curtailed. How far could this process go? At what point do I become only a line of thought-speech, without an environment of sensation and perception? What happens to the tracks when there is no longer ground to support the line? What happens to the spinning-top when only the axis is left? Where do thoughts come from? Upon what do they depend? Into how many worlds am I inserted? What is blindness?

'Can You Only Talk?'   *22 September 1984*

A lot of Thomas's behaviour at present with me consists of checking the various meanings which blindness has for our relationship. He understands most of these, but needs to check on various angles.

Today he was sitting on my knee at the table, colouring a dinosaur painting book. He asked if I would like to do some colouring. I said that I couldn't really do this because I couldn't see the edges. He commented, 'But I can colour because I can see the edges, because I'm not blind.'

I agreed. He went on colouring for a few moments and then looked up at me. I could feel his head turn around. 'Can you only talk?'

I laughed at this and said, 'I can talk and I can listen.'

'Yes!' he said brightly.

'And I can tickle.'

He agreed.

'And I can shout, listen.' I then gave an enormous bellow.

He was delighted with this and wanted me to shout again and again which I did. He joined in.

I summed up the meeting by saying, 'So, I can't see but I can talk and listen and tickle and shout.'

There was a pause while he seemed to consider the situation. He then made a suggestion, 'Look, Daddy. You can colour like this.' He put a crayon into my fingers, holding me by the hand and moving my hand backwards and forwards over the paper. I suggested that if he held my wrist he could move me around. I made rapid circular movements with the crayon and quickly shaded in most of the dinosaur. This pleased him very much, as it did me, and we repeated it several times.

Lizzie, eighteen months younger, is still almost entirely unaware of the significance of blindness. This morning I asked her to throw a tissue into the waste-paper basket. She ran across the room with it and called back to me, 'This one? Shall I throw it in here?' Thomas has reached the stage when he knows that he would have to come and get me, and make my hand touch the edge of the waste-paper basket.

Are Canada and Australia Places? *28 September 1984*

Looking back on the past few months, when I have been travelling to Canada and Australia, I do not have a very clear sense of having visited either place. It is true that here the people with whom I spoke had Canadian accents and there Australian, but that might happen in my own office in Birmingham. In my memory, I have a file of photographs of the Melbourne skyline, but I have not returned with this file updated. I did a tour by car of the eastern part of Lake Ontario, where the St Lawrence River begins, the area called One Thousand Islands. I remember the various comments made by my fellow-travellers inside the car. There was the time we stopped for an ice-cream and I walked over the gravelly car park. In what sense, however, can I say that these visits have added to my experience?

As the sighted traveller without a camera is to the sighted traveller with a camera, so am I to any sighted traveller. The sighted traveller with the camera is storing up visual memories, so that his or her present experiences can be prolonged, recalled and re-lived, shared with others and enjoyed again. As I, the blind traveller, sitting in the car, consider my sighted fellow-travellers, they are like someone who has a camera. They are continually filing away the memorable things they see, skylines, waterfalls, sunsets, islands and bridges, so that they will be able to live in them, talk about them, compare them with other places they have visited, cross-reference them and come back to them again and again. They will talk about where they have been, what their impressions were.

The sighted traveller with the camera says to a friend, 'Oh, but you'll have nothing to remember it by!' So the sighted people would say to the blind person (if it occurred to them to wonder what the experience was like), 'You'll have nothing to remember it by.' So it is that when I look back on the places I have visited in the past four years, my experience has not been enriched in any way commensurate with the effort involved in getting there. I have learned a great deal about those places, most of which I could have learned here but would not have bothered to. Having talked to people in their own homes in Houston about security problems in the American cities, I have stored up in my mind various impressions about life in America, but this hardly amounts to a visit to Houston. There is a certain immediacy about talking with people in their own city, in that the anecdotes are fresher, and you overhear their current conversations. But what to me are Houston, Ottawa, Melbourne?

Just as the blind get to know people by storing memories around the name of the person, so it is with cities. Around the cue-word 'Ottawa', I associate my memories of all the people I spoke with, the food I ate, the beds I slept in, and the hands I shook in Ottawa. That is what Ottawa means to me: that collection of memories of human contacts, so different from what is conjured up in the minds of sighted people by the names of cities. To the sighted, 'Sydney' conjures up a vision of the Harbour Bridge, 'Paris' the Eiffel Tower, and 'New York' the Empire State Building. In less dramatic and symbolic terms, the name of any town conjures up for a sighted person the images of what that town looks like. The blind person either has no such images at all, or projects in imagination images of what he or she thinks those cities would be like. We do not, however, learn from our own images, nor from our own memories, but only from our perceptions.

The result of all this in the experience of an adult recently blinded is a strange feeling that one has stopped accumulating experiences. Previously, one seemed always to be standing upon the edge of a line of experience which had been steadily expanding. It was like laying down a mosaic pavement. It was always possible to pause on the edge and look back at the pattern. As I look back now, I feel that the laying down of the mosaic ended in the summer of 1980. Since then I have been wandering over a trackless waste with very few co-ordinated and understood experiences to fill in the area between where I now am and the last line of the mosaic which I see far behind me. When you are travelling along a road punctuated by lots of houses or trees, you have a definite sense of speed and the passage of distance and time. When you start to travel through the trackless waste, through space or through the desert, through a featureless world, you lose that sense. Vast spaces seem small; sometimes small spaces seem vast. This is aggravated by the lack of any succession of day or night, and the absence of any vivid realization of the passage of the seasons. The days grow colder but not shorter, there is no question of the autumn leaves this year being more beautiful, more memorable, than the lovely autumn of several years ago. Experience has lost its punctuation marks.

The way a blind adult recollects experience is rather like the way any adult recollects his or her experience from infancy. Many adults, when trying to remember their childhood, search for visual images of the sort that they would now be able to collect if they were in those places, e.g. the appearance of furniture or of the interior of rooms, the layout of the backyard or the line of shops near the house. The point is, however, that to the young child things did not look like that, and thus could not be stored in a form which the adult can recollect or can recognize as being similar to more recently stored images. Now and again, back and beyond the occasional visual inspiration, lies something deeper which can be called body memory. This is not so much memory of what things looked like, but recollection of how things felt. The most vivid of these are usually not of a specific event but of some regular happening. They are difficult to distinguish from the moments of empathy which an adult has with a child experiencing the same thing.

So it is with the memories of the blind adult. They focus upon what one's body experienced, or underwent. This is quite different from visual memory, because your body does not feel what your eye sees.

So my memories of Melbourne consist of the innumerable car journeys from place to place, and the different textures of this seat belt and that car upholstery. From such and such a city I remember the discomfort of standing in the cold wind, from another the stiffness of sitting for hours in the same chair, from another the comfort of the smooth cool tiles in the bathroom. My memory is like the memory of a snail. My body can recollect the narrow little strip of ground over which I have passed, and it consists of tiny details, so tiny as to be irrelevant from the point of view of the cat and the dog. Here the footpath goes up slightly, there is a nick in the kerb, this telephone pole has a metal plate screwed to it but this other one is smooth.

This route, like the path of a snail, is what I know about my walk from home to the office. It is not exactly going from one place to another place through some intermediate places. When I try to visualize my route, what I do is to anticipate the sensations which my body will have at various times (that is, places) along that route. Here I will be guided by something which I will pass on my left, later on it will be something on my right. What lies more than two or three feet away on either side of that trail means nothing to me. It is not part of my experience, except when it comes home to me in traffic noise or birdsong. My place is known to me by the soles of my feet and by the tip of my cane.

A Bend in the Tunnel   *29 September 1984*

I can now reflect upon the meaning of the whole Australian experience. I have turned a corner in the tunnel. So far, there has been light at the end. True, I have been travelling away from that light, deeper and deeper from it; nevertheless, the light has been there, behind me. It has been an ever-diminishing pinpoint, yet its presence has served to orientate and guide. At least, there was some point of definition in the past from which I was receding. It has been like a bright star from which my spacecraft has been moving further and further away, but I only know this because of the star, which fixes a point from which my position becomes more and more remote.

Going back to the image of the tunnel, I have turned a corner. The pinpoint of light seems to have vanished.

The light at the end of the tunnel consisted of my memories of my forty-five years of sighted life. This seems to fall into two sections. There are twenty-four years (1935–59) spent in Australia. Then there are twenty-one years (1959–80) spent in England, fourteen of them in Birmingham. The part of the light represented by my years in Birmingham has gradually had superimposed upon it memories from my years of blindness. There are now many journeys which I can make by car through the streets of Birmingham, along familiar routes, and I can tell where I am by the turns and twists of the car. I am like a dog, asleep on the back seat, that wakes up a block or two from home. He knows in his body those familiar final twists and turns of the car. These memories have, to some extent, taken the place of the visual memories of the streets. Of course, it is true that I am still much better off in Birmingham than I would be in any other city, because there is still so much of my blind experience which is enriched by my sighted memories. So, for example, I still see the University clock tower, Big Joe, in my imagination. This helps to fill out my environment and to know where I am. The first twenty-four years are, however, entirely light. There had been no opportunity, apart from the visit to Melbourne in 1980 when I was partially sighted, to superimpose upon that visual layer a gradual re-adjustment of blind memories. Between me and that sighted past there has now built up a sort of protective wall. When I think of Australia now, it not only conjures up visions of dazzling, golden beaches, swaying eucalyptus forests, and the dry hillsides with their rocky outcrops, but also the bumpiness of the car rides, the wheezing from room to room, the feel of the handrails at Melbourne Zoo, and the fragrance of the bush.

There are parts of my twenty-one years of sighted English experience which are still brightly lit. The light seems to fall on all the places which I have not revisited as a blind person. Every time I do revisit one of these places, it comes home to me with a sense of loss that now, instead of accumulating further visual images, bringing up to date the memories I have, making a mental note of changes, and finding out what lay beyond the corner I had not had time to visit previously, I have to start again, helped to some extent by the visual memories, but knowing the city now as part of a different world. So my entire visual stock of knowledge is receding into the past, becoming less useful, less relevant to me, less accurate. It is the dramatic realization of the remoteness of that visual past brought on by the Melbourne visit which I am referring to as turning the corner in a tunnel. Just as the disappearance of the final speck of light means that I have to find new ways of orientating myself in space, so it also means that I must find new ways of orientating myself within my life span. I am now in blind time, not sighted time.

What is the meaning of blindness? It is strange that after four years of being registered, and two years of total blindness, I am still seeking to understand this question.

7

Beyond Feelings

Winter 1984

Your Image on the Far Side   *13 October 1984*

Last night Marilyn and I were talking about whether or not it would have
made a difference to my feelings about Thomas and Elizabeth if I had
ever seen them. Is the fact that I have never seen them going to be a
permanent loss in my relationship with them? Does it matter that they
belong entirely to my second life, my blind life?

It is true that Imogen bridges both lives. She was seven when I lost
my sight; now she is eleven. Is it not possible, however, that Imogen will
remain in my imagination permanently fixed at the age of seven, while
Marilyn will always remain young and beautiful?

This is relevant to the experience of blindness as a journey into a dark
tunnel. The receding faces of Imogen and Marilyn form a sort of fixed
light at the far end, behind me. This provides a point of reference from
which I can judge my continued travelling on through the tunnel. In a
way, this serves to exaggerate the time I have spent in the tunnel, by
providing a point of orientation which makes me aware of the continual
recessions of the light. It is as if during the first part of a journey through
space the voyagers are aware of the speed with which they are parting
from the still visible earth, but once out in the black vastness of space,
there is no longer the same sense of speed, or time. As long as there is a
receding image, one is still aware of departing.

On the other hand, the element of fixation in this, that you go on
thinking of the person as he or she was years ago, makes time less real.
You have a sense of not having travelled on in your relationships. There

is conflict between the timeless, fixated image of not travelling on, and (on the other hand) the sharpened sense of distance, that one is travelling on, further and further, all the time. This conflict helps me to understand the strange poignancy and confusion which I feel in the presence of loved people whom once I saw but now no longer see. This would also explain my distress in meeting my Australian relatives, especially my parents, in the summer.

This is a good example of what the psychologists call 'cognitive dissonance'. There is discomfort because you are aware of holding two opinions or beliefs which are contradictory. First, I believe that I know what you look like. I have your image in my mind's eye as I speak with you now. Thus, although I am blind, nothing has changed. I have not changed. You have not changed. I can still relate to you through the mediation provided by that visual image, which is in my memory. Secondly, I know that between that visual memory which mediates between us and my actual present life there is a deep, black river of time, flooding the banks of my consciousness, growing ever wider and stronger, carrying us apart. Your image is there, on the far side, always receding and now totally inaccessible. I have changed. You have changed. Everything is changed. There is a conflict between these two beliefs.

The discomfort of this contradiction can make you feel a little uneasy, or it can become quite painful. It can be relieved in various ways. I may try to turn my back upon your image as it glows brightly on the far side of the floor. Now I can try to reconstruct my relationship to you on a completely new basis, on this side, where we are now. On the other hand, I may be tempted to linger in the past, to indulge in the contemplation of your remembered image, and to have it always before me, so that always speaking with you I am deliberately conversing through that loved image. In the first case, I try to abolish the past. In the second, I live in the past.

In my relationship with Thomas and Lizzie I am not aware of this particular conflict. Rather, I have been marginalized as a father. My interaction with them is now severely limited, and I am not the sort of father that I would like to be. Nevertheless, in their presence I do not experience that strange sense of baffled shock that I sometimes feel with Imogen and Marilyn, and particularly with my parents. Thomas and Lizzie are entirely children of my blindness. They are habituated there, and so my relationship with them is not inhibited by visual memories from the past. It develops entirely along the lines of a non-visual relationship. Do I, then, experience 'growing old together' with Thomas and Lizzie? Is there a common participation in a maturing pattern of experience? Are we really together, sharing this time and space? The answer is yes. The base may be narrow, but the shared community is there. With Imogen and Marilyn, I feel less certain.

With a loved woman, so much of the experience of growing older together lies in witnessing the work of time. Perhaps in the case of a child who is becoming an adolescent, it lies in witnessing the growing up process. I want to know how that childlike face and figure are being transformed into those of a young woman. Would it be different with a son?

My relationship with the younger children has elements of role alienation (loss of fatherhood) but my relationship with Imogen and Marilyn has traces of cognitive conflict (relating past to present).

This applies to my relationship with myself. I know what I looked like because of memories of photographs and seeing myself in the mirror. Oddly enough, many of the photographs which I remember most vividly are not recent, but were taken years ago, and have stuck in my mind. So I know that my memories of myself are already out of date, and the strange thing is that I have no way of updating them. This means that I have a sense of cognitive dissonance when I think about myself. On the one hand, I know that I am such and such a person, with certain features. On the other hand, I know myself as someone who probably no longer looks like that, and I cannot witness the work of time upon my own face. How can I grow old together even with myself?

I have become separated from my own shadow, as in the cartoons. A quivering image of myself is left behind, while the real me has been blown away by a sudden explosion, which has split me into two images. Each one has a different expression and posture, and is doing different things. I have a double relationship with myself.

Should I forget all about my old, sighted appearance? Should I now try to get to know myself again entirely on the basis of non-visual data? That is clearly inevitable. What will become, then, of those forty-five years of being a sighted self?

This must be part of the reason why it was so painful returning to Australia, because I was confronted by the first twenty-four years, the childhood and youth of that sighted self, from whom I have now become divided because I am plunged into different ways of knowing my present self.

Getting Lost   *8 November 1984*

I think it is David Scott Blackhall, in his autobiography *The Way I See Things*, who remarks how annoying he found it when people refused to answer his question about where he was and insisted on asking him where he was trying to get to. I share this experience.

Going home the other night I was turned out of my way by some construction work on one of the footpaths. By mistake I turned along a side street, and after a block or so, when I realized I had made a mistake somewhere, I was not sure exactly where I was. There were some chaps working on a car parked on the roadside. 'Excuse me,' I said. 'Could you tell me please where I am? What is the name of this street?'

The man replied, 'Where are you trying to get to?'

With what I hoped was a good-humoured laugh, I said, 'Never mind about that, just tell me, please, what street this is?'

'This is Alton Road. You usually go up Bournbrook Road don't you? It's just a block further along.'

I thanked him, and explained that I needed now to know exactly whereabouts in Alton Road I was so that I could get to Bournbrook Road. 'Which *side* of Alton Road am I on? If I face that way, am I looking towards Bristol Road or is it the other way?'

'You live high up Bournbrook Road, don't you? Well, if you take the next to the left you'll be OK.'

But which way is 'left'? Does he mean me to cross the road or to stay on this side? At this point, the blind and the sighted enter into mutual bafflement.

When sighted people are lost, what matters to them is not where they are, but where they are going. When they are told that the building they are looking for lies in a certain direction, they are no longer lost. A sighted person is lost in the sense that he or she does not know where a particular building is. Sighted people are never lost with respect to what street they are actually in; they just look at the street sign on the corner of the block. It is their direction they have lost, rather than their position. The blind person lost has neither direction nor position. The blind person needs position in order to discover direction. This is such a profound lostness that most sighted people find it difficult to imagine.

Taxis   *10 November 1984*

Sighted people often help me to hail taxis. I can't help noticing how frequently my new-found friend will not only lead me over the road to the taxi, but will give the taxi driver instructions. As we are walking along towards the taxi rank, my guide will ask me where I am going. Then, when he has got me into the taxi, making sure that I do not bang my head, he will then relay these directions to the driver.

The sighted person is caring for me. He is looking after me. The relationship of caring makes him feel that he is an adult and I am a child. If you were putting a child into a taxi, you would try to find out from the child exactly where he lived or where he thought he was going. You would not leave it to the child to negotiate with the taxi driver. You would make sure that the driver had absorbed this information and fully understood it before allowing the child to pass out of your care and be driven away. So it is between sighted and blind people.

'Are You Gobbling Up?'   *11 December 1984*

Thomas is very interested in how I know things, and what the extent and detail of my knowledge is. At breakfast this morning I said, 'Now you are gobbling up! That's a good boy.'

He said. 'How do you know?'

'I can hear you, and I can feel you.' I had stretched out my hand and placed it on his back, and could feel his body vibrating as he ate.

He moved away a little and ate more quietly, asking 'Can you still hear me? Am I gobbling now?'

'Yes, I can still hear you.'

Eating even more quietly, he inquired again.

'No,' I replied. 'I can't hear you now. Are you gobbling up?'

'Yes,' he replied cheerfully and began to eat vigorously once more. He had discovered the limit.

Whilst getting dressed upstairs, in my presence, he said to Marilyn, 'When I'm a lot older, say, about ten, will Daddy's eyes have got better?'

Marilyn replied, 'No, Thomas, they won't have got better.'

'Will they get better after a long, long, long time?'

'No, dear, they'll never get better.'

'Oh.'

Hospital   *13 December 1984*

I spent ten days in hospital. I was in a small, two-bed ward, just off the main ward, which had about twenty beds in it. The day room, where the telephone was, was at the far end of the main ward. To get to the telephone, I had to walk along the aisle down the middle of the main ward, with a line of beds on either side.

The first time I made this journey, it was a nightmare. It was the nearest thing to running the gauntlet I have ever experienced. I was a sensation. With my white cane, I commanded the attention of every eye. Every conversation stopped. Every man in the ward called out advice. 'Left a little! Right a little! Watch out, mate! Now you are OK, mate! Straight ahead and you'll be all right. Watch out for the trolley! On you go! Now stop a bit.' I was thoroughly confused by all this and found it impossible to concentrate.

When I got to the end of the ward, I stopped and asked one of the men who had been giving me this friendly encouragement to read to me a telephone number, which was written on a piece of paper. A young lad came across and read it. I memorized it, thanked him and went on my way. I heard an older man say to this lad, 'You'd better go after him and make sure he's OK.' A moment later, pattering feet behind me, and a hand came on my arm. I turned round and said rather bluntly but with a smile, 'What do you want?'

The lad laughed, and, slightly embarrassed, replied, 'I've just come to make sure that you didn't, er, bump into the door.'

I replied, 'Well, thank you very much, but in helping me in that way, you've made me forget the telephone number.'

He laughed at this, and I pulled the piece of paper out of my pocket. 'Now, what was it?'

He read it for me and I set off again. From behind, he shouted out, 'Left a little, watch out, now you're OK, it's straight ahead.'

Turning around I said, 'Ssssh – you'll make me forget it again!'

'Sorry,' he called, as I found the door to the day room, went through and made my call.

The return trip was just as bad. Once again, every man in the place was helping me. The air was thick with cries of 'Left a little, right a little, back a little.' I felt unable to ignore these calls, and was turning from left to right, like Prince Philip at an exhibition, thanking this man and that man, saying hello and goodbye, assuring them that I was all right, in the midst of which it was quite impossible to concentrate and I was in real danger of walking into a trolley. When I got back to my own little room, I found that my hands were moist with perspiration, my heart was beating with excitement, and I felt completely exhausted. I was overcome with the effort and with the embarrassment.

From then on, I made my telephone calls late at night when everyone was asleep. It was perfectly simple to walk down the aisle, touching lightly the end of an occasional bed just to make sure I was going straight. I never had the slightest difficulty in finding the phone, and I never bumped into anything, provided all the men were asleep. It is these offers of help which really disable me.

An End of Mourning   *30 January 1985*

I was on my way home one evening last November. I was standing at
the traffic lights on the Bristol Road waiting for the bleeps. I suddenly
became aware of the contrast between what I must have looked like and
what I felt like. All these people rushing past in their cars must be
thinking, 'Gosh. There's a blind man. I hope he doesn't step out in front
of me. I wonder if he'll be all right. Perhaps I should slow down or see
if he needs help. I wonder why he hasn't got a dog.'

On the inside, however, I felt light-hearted, competent, in a situation
I knew I could handle. The noise of the traffic, coming from either
direction, was full and rich, the peripheral sounds made by people
walking on the footpath, louder on this side of the road, fainter on the
other side, and all of the other echoes and contours made up that
acoustic shape which I call the Bristol Road. In a few moments the noise
of the traffic would change. Instead of the present movement of ap-
proaching and departing rushes of sound there would be the purring of
engines idling on either side. Between would be a silent space. I would
lean forward, stretch out my white cane to its full length, tap it briskly
first on one side of me and then on the other, so announcing my intention
to cross (if anyone could have doubted it) and would then step boldly
out into that silent space. I would walk across the road rapidly, strike
the far kerb with my cane, and step up on to the footpath, turning round
briefly to wave at the imagined drivers before coming to rest against the
iron pickets of the fence. By now, behind me, the gap would have closed,
and the roaring passage of movement from both sides would have
flooded the place through which I had passed. I had made it, one more
time.

It struck me, however, as I stood waiting for the bleeps, that what to
me was a perfectly normal, full and informative environment, telling me
everything I needed for a safe crossing, must look very different to the
motorist. The thought went through my mind, 'They think I'm blind,
but I'm not!' What I meant to think was, 'They think I'm ignorant and
helpless, that I don't really know where I am and that I will probably do
something silly and dangerous to myself or to them. But I am probably
as safe as the average sighted pedestrian at this crossing.'

Looking back now, I think that this was the first time I had a feeling
of calmness and confidence as a blind person in a blind person's world,
in which I could move reasonably safely, and easily. Now that a satisfac-
tory Christmas is behind me, I feel more clearly than before that the
Australian experience of last summer was a turning-point, if not a

breaking-point, in my period of mourning over the loss of sight. I am sometimes still afflicted by a sharp sense of grief and loss, particularly in the presence of the children, but on the whole I am calmer. Life has become bearable, I am more or less in control of my situation and of my work and of my feelings about it. I daresay that many of these feelings will recur, and that I shall lapse into mourning again and again. Nevertheless, the basic period of mourning is over.

It has taken four-and-a-half years to reach this point. On the radio programme *In Touch* the other day someone was speaking of her own period of mourning for the loss of sight. With an apologetic laugh, she remarked that it had taken a full fortnight. I am amazed at how some people seem to be able to adjust so quickly, so vigorously. For me, it has been like a long, slow and lingering death.

Feeling Beyond Feelings   *3 February 1985*

I seem to be all right as long as I take the initiative. The children were given a large construction set for Christmas. The nuts and bolts were as big as adults' fingers. The plastic building strips were from eight to eighteen inches long. It was a primitive, childlike sort of thing, quite easy for a blind person to handle. Lego, on the other hand, is too tiny and complicated.

A few weeks ago, Thomas and I had a splendid time playing with this construction set on a Saturday morning. We made a space gun, and then a high chair for Teddy. It was on wheels and everything. It was by far the best playtime I have ever had with him. I was doing something, and we were doing it together. Most of the time, I am merely present while things are being done. Even when we do things together, it is often individually but simultaneously, like eating, which we do at the same time, but separately. The fun about building with the construction set was that it was reciprocal.

Today was rather different. An old and much-loved friend of the family came with late Christmas presents. There were a series of little plastic tubes of foam rubber which turned into animal shapes when placed in warm water. The children loved them. There were shrieks of delight from the bathroom as each new animal wiggled into life.

Next, there were a couple of super mobiles, including a clown. You had to hang various rings, bangles and performing animals over his hands and feet.

The next morning I woke feeling remote and sleepy. During the morning, a little boy came to play with Thomas and Lizzie. This situation is always rather difficult, because I never know exactly what they are doing. I miss the reactions and the interreactions. It is so hard to tell what the one who isn't shouting at the moment is doing. I put on a record, and went into the dining room to listen on the extension speakers. I had to stand up and lean against the wall to keep myself awake. Waves of sleep passed over me and in the end I went upstairs to lie down. I switched myself off for about three-quarters of an hour.

I rallied for lunch, but afterwards Thomas asked me to play with the clown mobile. I had a sinking feeling that this would be very difficult, but I badly wanted to try. I allowed him to lead me into the living room and when I sat down he put the mobile into my hands. It was a mass of shapes and string. After some exploration, I discovered what must have been the peaked hat of the clown. He seemed to be standing on one leg, with the second leg kicking in the air. He was running, Thomas said. I held the clown in an upright position while Thomas began to decorate him with the bits and pieces of the mobile.

During this time, spasms rather than waves of sleep were flicking through my brain. I felt more and more remote. Coming into the room, Marilyn was rather alarmed when she saw me, and urged me to go into the office. Most reluctantly, I took her advice, and set out with a heavy heart. Withdrawal, whether internal or external, was my only form of defence.

Even walking into work I felt groggy, and as soon as I dropped into my comfortable office chair I fell into a dazed, dopey sort of fitful sleep which lasted for nearly three hours. I was just beginning to come round, and get my cassettes organized on the desk to begin work when Marilyn phoned.

It was very much like being drugged. Whilst playing with the mobile, I felt the way you do when you have just had the anaesthetic before an operation. You start to feel sleep creeping over you. What I felt was not as irresistible as that, of course, otherwise I would have fallen over. Nevertheless, it was that kind of thing.

This must be a protection against an unbearable situation. I hear the children and everyone else whooping with delight, making comments, and it is as if the knowledge which I do have mocks the knowledge which I don't have, while the poignancy of that contrast makes me want to have no more knowledge at all.

The visit of the old friend was certainly another factor. She played so happily with the children, and with such imagination. She pointed things out, oohed and ahed as things were opened, and sat down to look at the pop-up book. This detailed exchange of playful interludes somehow made me more sharply aware of my own difficulties in playing with the children, and of the lack of finesse and detail which has blurred my play with them. I have always had a particular love for the minute details of children's behaviour.

The strange thing is that I would not describe my reaction as being an emotion. Similarly, as I have already learned, the depression associated with blindness is not a feeling. In the situation I am describing I do not actually feel sad, and I certainly have no feelings of bitterness. When I think of my relationship with Imogen when she was two or three, and how we used to play together for hours, and I compare it with my present habits of play with Thomas and Lizzie, I do have an emotion. It is hard to say what that emotion is. Is it possible to be in the grip of an emotion so strong and so close that one cannot put a name to it? Is it possible that we can only name our milder feelings? Does emotion, like light, dazzle us when it becomes too intense? The best I can do is to say that it is a poignant sense of loss. There is also a sense of longing for a relationship, for an experience, and perhaps some panic at the thought that this is now all passing me by and these golden years of children's play will never be recovered.

Then it seems to me that I have lost Imogen, my daughter from my former marriage, in one way and I am losing these present children in a different way.

In this situation I don't, however, feel at all tearful, and I am not aware of anger, self-pity or pathos. It is rather as if an intention has taken the place of a feeling. The intention is to withdraw. The emotional life is no longer experienced as content (that is, as an emotion having the identifiable content of anger, sadness, and so on) but as a sort of numbness of recoil. I seek refuge in sleep, or sleep seeks to inhabit me.

As soon as I am out of the presence of the children and in a position to give in to these feelings, I do become conscious of a certain desolation, but mainly of a sort of incapacity, an inability to think or act, a confusion or drifting away, together with a sense of bodily comfort as sleep swamps me.

This seems to take several hours to work through. Sometimes it is after the children have had their baths and gone to bed that I feel better. I may be in the office, and not even be thinking of going home yet, but I somehow improve as if a demand has been lifted. Sometimes the turning-point comes even earlier, when I know that the regular routine of the evening, the bathing and changing, the goodnight ritual has begun. I take part in this, quite often and quite successfully. It is as if I know that playtime is now over, and a sequence has begun which I can handle.

It is only sitting down now and thinking about it that I notice these apparent regularities.

A Secret Door   *4 February 1985*

Trying to work in my office one weekend I fell into a heavy, depressed sleep, as if drugged. I had a vivid dream about the office. The room was full of light. I noticed that I had not closed the office door. People were walking to and fro in the corridor, and I realized that they might have seen me there, fast asleep in my chair. All of this was in the dream. Perhaps I was half awake? There was a wardrobe with a light in it. I was feeling for the light, groping for the switch. When the light was on, it was so intensely bright that every detail in the wardrobe stood out. The clothes hanging on hooks appeared in brilliant detail against the clear, cream wall. When I gazed around the room, the illumination seemed to be patchy and to bring to my attention details I had never noticed before. What was this? A door. An internal door, leading perhaps to the next office. It is a painted, wooden door, of the old-fashioned type, with carved, oblong panels and a round, domestic-type knob. It is a rich, chocolate brown against the surrounding cream wall. I look at this door with amazement, wondering how it could be that, in all my feeling round this room and in my belief that I knew every nook and cranny of it, I had never noticed it. Then I woke up.

Upon awakening, this dream struck me as strange and deeply moving. But I could not tell why. It is about privacy, and the loss of privacy, enclosures, including three doors, one open, one through which I can half go (the wardrobe door) and the secret door. The dream is about the relationships between various kinds of interiors. These interiors are related in different ways to the world, and the dream describes the various kinds of frustrations and possibilities which blindness, the necessary avenue of communication between my interior and the world, poses. There is a strange hope in the mysterious, tightly closed but previously unnoticed door. There is always more to a familiar place than you realize. In the most intimately loved situation, if you look closely, there is often another door.

A Body without a World and a   *5 February 1985*
World without a Body

Clive Inman, after his road accident, spent six months in hospital and a further six months or so undergoing physiotherapy. He can now walk again, and drive his car, but he has no sensation of heat or cold in his body below his neck except in one or two fingers. He told me the other day that he can only tell when he is hot by noticing whether he is sweating. If he is shivering, then he knows he must be cold. I pointed out that sometimes his palms would be sweaty or clammy when he was nervous, so how would he know whether it was nervousness or heat? Clive replied that his psyche informed him when he was nervous, but his psyche did not inform him when his body was hot. He agreed, however, that there might well be times when one would notice that one's palms were sweating, and would think 'Goodness! I *must* be nervous.' In such a situation, where the symptom drew attention to the state, he might not know which state the symptom indicated.

I asked Clive whether he did not feel that he was no longer living in that part of his body which is below his neck. He agreed that often he did have a very strange feeling of being disassociated from his own body.

Clive's situation is the opposite to my own. I, as a blind person, tend to be enclosed within my body, to be conscious primarily of it, and to be cut off from the world. He, on the other hand, is cut off from his body. He has perfect senses, and knows just what he wants his body to do in the world, but his body will not do it. My body will do perfectly well what I want it to do in the world, but it has no world within which to do it. In the early stages of his physiotherapy, he could not walk but he knew exactly where he wanted to walk. I can walk perfectly, but I do not know where to walk. I have no world to walk in; he had no body to walk with.

Snow   *16 February 1985*

Many sighted people express concern about how I manage in the snow. It is true that snow creates a considerable problem for blind people. There is a saying: snow is the blind person's fog.

Most sighted people have some difficulty in realizing the nature of my problem. They tend to assume that I will be 'slipping and sliding'. In other words, they attribute to me the same difficulty which they are having in the snow, on the assumption that if they are slipping and sliding I must be slipping and sliding even more.

My problem is not instability but mobility. It is not that I become unsure of my footing, but I become unsure about where I am going. What I suffer in the snow is a loss of knowledge. All my familiar points and markings, the different grades and textures of grass, gravel, asphalt and concrete are obliterated. If the snow is deep enough to cover the kerbs, then I really have a problem, because I cannot tell one block from the next, or the road from the footpath. I explain to people that I have good, solid boots, I have never slipped yet and am perfectly steady on my feet. The problem, I explain, is that I cannot tell my route.

Sighted people find it difficult to realize that, for a blind person, the body itself has become the organ of sense. Apart from the white cane, and the sounds from the environment, the body's knowledge of its surroundings does not exceed its own dimensions. This is such a curious position to be in, such a strange kind of reality for the body in the world, that the sighted can hardly grasp it.

What Do Numbers Look Like?   *25 February 1985*

Today I could not remember which way the arabic number three points. I had to trace it with my finger in the air, one, two, three. Now I remember. It points to the left. If it points to the right, it is a bit like the letter E. Marilyn was with me, and was surprised to find that such a deeply ingrained image could be partially lost.

I also had to ask her whether the border which goes around the edge of a tablecloth or a board is spelt 'border' or 'boarder'. I think I was confused about the board around which there is a border. This illustrates how much the ability to spell is based upon visual images.

Bar Talk   *8 March 1985*

When I was sighted, I often used to have a drink and a sandwich in the bar in Staff House. Even if I went in by myself, I would seldom be alone for long. I would see somebody I knew, or thought I knew, or pretended I knew. There would be a slight nod, a flicker of a smile, and I would find myself having a chat with somebody.

All this has changed. I have to wait until someone approaches me, or I have to recognize the voice of somebody I know. In a crowded bar, that is not easy. Moreover, the people whose voices I know well enough to recognize in that situation, are people I know very well indeed, and not the casual acquaintances whom I would have met in previous days. I can no longer introduce myself to strangers, because blindness has taken from me all of the preliminary steps, the little acknowledgements, the half-questioning, tentative approaches.

These days, I often go into the bar, stand there drinking my pint, wondering whether anyone will speak to me. Often, nobody does. The strange thing is that, as I am leaving, and am taking the eight or ten steps from the bar to the door of the room, I am suddenly approached by all manner of people, hands stretch out, concerned voices ask if I am all right, and quite often I find that amongst them there are people who know me. Maybe they hadn't noticed me at the bar. Maybe they had been engaged in their own conversations. Maybe they thought I wanted to drink alone. The irony of it is that now I am besieged with offers of help which I don't need, while previously, when any offer of social converse would have been gladly accepted, I was left to myself.

One of the problems is that in the bar at Staff House, people do not tend to know each other's names. One can often go in there, find half a dozen people you know or have seen on the campus, but no one whose name you know. For me, knowledge of the names is the vehicle of social mobility. I travel on people's elbows and on people's names.

Moreover, when I had sight, of ten conversations I might have had in the bar, seven or eight would have been initiated by me. The change enforced upon my personality is thus more severe than would have been the case had I been a shy and retiring person. What to do about it? I must come to the sad conclusion that there is little point in dropping into the bar for the casual drink. I must always go accompanied. I must make sure by ringing round my friends beforehand that I always meet someone who is expecting me. I know what will happen next; I will be ringing round, but no one will ring me. Why not? Because the practice is not to ring round in that way, but just to drop in at the bar and have a drink on the off-chance that there will be someone there you know. The other problem is that people will think I am seeking help in getting to the bar itself. I will have offers of coming to my room and escorting me. It is so hard to help people to see that physical mobility is no problem. What worries me is social mobility.

People not Photographs   *9 March 1985*

Blind people do not make very good photographers. They have no way of freezing the present moment, of encapsulating the flow of a relationship within a little, static frame. They live in a world of speech, of process and of movement.

Perhaps this means that we, who are blind, ought to be better listeners. This is not because, being unable to see, we have no alternative to listening. That would be a mere deficiency-motive, an incentive provided by a loss. The blind person's ability to listen is created by the way in which other people are experienced. He or she has less control over the past, less opportunity to fixate the past, and more openness to the impact of a present relationship. The fact that human beings are so ephemeral to the blind person, that they appear to come and go, means that the presence of another human being is a very distinct mark of present experience. Because the human relationships of blind people are presented to them in a uniquely forceful and striking manner, they have a quality of 'presence'. The blind experience friendship as a gift, and a gift given now.

A Nocturnal Animal   *10 March 1985*

My efforts to understand the impact of blindness upon my life have taken a new twist. Yesterday I had a very happy day with the family. Imogen was here for the weekend, and after breakfast all the children played Ludo with me. Some visitors arrived in the middle of the morning and stayed for lunch. In the afternoon Marilyn and I took the children in the car to a playground. I pushed them on the swings and turned the big wheel around while they sat on it. By four o'clock when we were coming home, I became aware of being rather tense. By bathtime, an hour later, the tension had increased and during the evening meal, between six and half past, I was feeling I could not go on much longer. Marilyn, noticing that I was becoming withdrawn, suggested that I should try to do some work upstairs. I did not feel sleepy, but by half-past seven I was, in fact, fast asleep and did not wake for three hours. The house was silent, the children were in bed, and I felt much better. What had gone wrong with the day? Why had I gone like this after such a happy time?

The tension is not necessarily associated with depression, although it can be triggered by depression. It leads to an absence of feeling and movement, a sort of catatonic state. It also takes longer to come out of the situation when it is associated with depression.

What happened yesterday seems to be independent both of happiness and of depression. It is some kind of cognitive state.

The role of sleep is also different. When the tension is associated with depression, I am overcome by a desire, perhaps a need, to sleep. On this occasion I did not feel sleepy during the day, and when I went to my study about seven in the evening, it was with the intention of working, not sleeping. I found that I could not work, because I needed an item of information which was only available in my office. I could not go on with the micro-cassette dictation I was doing, and, in the end, I lay down and went to sleep because I had run out of things to do. Sleep is a very acceptable substitute for work, but I was not actually overcome by irresistible waves of sleep.

Although my best policy is still to take the initiative and in that way to fend off the feelings of passivity and nonentity which bring on the depression, there remains nevertheless a strange kind of cognitive or psychological exhaustion which overcomes me, in spite of happiness. What is this?

Noise may be a factor. It is natural enough that I have become sensitive to noise. It certainly was rather a noisy day. Two older children were having a disco upstairs. Two younger boys were enjoying an exciting game of 'He-man' in my study. The radio was on downstairs, and a group of younger children were racing around everywhere. The whole house was gradually strewn with toys, despite the best efforts of hard-pressed adults to tidy up, so that in the end I could hardly take a step unless I cleared the ground in front of me, like some sacred ritual. All that makes me feel bombarded; I cannot respond even though the environment is calling out to me. This gives a sense of remoteness.

At work, I can control the bombardment, at least to some extent, by creating a predictable day. I have my hand on the tap, so to speak, and can increase or decrease the flow, more or less as I wish. I can bring the interview to an end. Even if I am stuck in a seminar or a committee, I know that it will finish in an hour or so. At home it is different.

Any normal adult would feel somewhat similar in circumstances like these. The children really wear Marilyn out, and would wear anyone out. As far as I can tell, however, my experience is not quite like this. It did not affect me like this before I lost my sight. It is quite different now. The sense of recoil, of numbness is greater, and there is this strange feeling that one is becoming more and more unreal.

Can it be that I have become a sort of nocturnal animal? When such a creature is forced to remain up and to mix all day, under the bright light, with the daylight animals, its senses become hounded until it longs for the stillness and silence of a retreat where it can recover. In my case, the metaphor breaks down, because there is no particular time of night. There is no night-time just as there is no day-time.

Is there any more to this than metaphor? Am I becoming a creature of the night? Am I not close to dreams? Does not blindness give me an affinity with darkness? If the sun is the symbol of consciousness then the moon represents the magical sources of our deeper life. Not only am I cut off from the physical sun, but less tolerant of consciousness unless it is frequently bathed in the mysterious energies of its opposite.

8

Still Looking

Spring 1985

The Meaning of Black Wholes   11 *March 1985*

I am struck by the stoicism in many of the autobiographies of blind people which I have read. An outstanding example is the autobiography of the war-wounded hero Sir Michael Ansell whose book is appropriately called *Soldier On*. Sir Michael Ansell lost his sight in an unfortunate misunderstanding during the confused withdrawal of the British Expeditionary Force before the expanding German onslaught in 1940. He and his companions were sheltering in a barn when they were attacked by a group of British soldiers who thought that they were Germans. The rest of the book tells of the influence of this remarkable man in British showjumping, including his work in creating the 'Horse of the Year Show' and as the trainer of the British team for the Equestrian Olympics. Even when he lost his first wife, through cancer, and his second wife, who was tragically killed in a road accident, the story continues in the same completely matter-of-fact way. There is not a trace of self-pity or even of self-analysis in the whole book.

I cannot write a stoical or a matter-of-fact book; I have to write in my own way, trying to understand what is happening to me. This must include some effort to understand blindness itself, as well as my own blindness. In seeking understanding, I am seeking for meaning. This statement is already made in faith. I am already committed to the value that a unified life is superior to a fragmented life, and a full meaning is better than a partial one. Of course, the quest for full significance and for complete integration will never be ended. It will never be a finished product. Nevertheless, the quest remains worthwhile. I will be all the more sane if I have been able to accept, to include, to harmonize more and more of my experience.

When I speak of seeking understanding, I am thinking of faith *in search of* understanding. This is why, for me, there can be no stoical resignation before an inscrutable destiny, no gritting of the teeth, no acceptance, however courageous, of a meaningless destiny.

This is the sense in which, in my opinion, it would not be a Christian act to accept blindness, or try to go on as if it had not happened, or to defy it through mere courage, although I cannot but have the deepest respect for those noble blind people who have responded in those ways. My desire for coherence, a desire which in my case has taken the Christian form, impels me to probe the experience, to grapple with it, to strip off layer after layer from it, to find meaning within it and to relate that meaning to the other parts or aspects of living.

This approach does not suggest that I would look for any specific meaning peculiar to blindness itself as if 'the blindness was sent for a reason' or as if I would be interested in the answer to the question 'Why did this happen to me?' Since the meaning which I seek will be coherent, it will lie in the wholeness. Blindness is a part of my life, and I must try to understand its particular characteristics so that I can be faithful in this part. I must, however, never forget that blindness is only a part. My overriding attempt must be to have the courage to be faithful as a whole, that is as a person in whose life this is one aspect amongst many others. Taking the thought still further, my own life is but a part of a still larger whole, and if I am coherent with that larger whole, I will again be a whole myself, but at a more universal level. This is part of what I understand communion with God to mean.

In the attempt to integrate one's life around a meaning, one of the dangers which one faces is reduction. One tends to set up a meaning-making machine, like a sausage-making machine, so that no matter what kind of experiences you pour in one end, exactly the same kind of sausages or meanings come out the other end. Inconsistencies are excluded, and only the homogeneous is retained. The result is a strong identity but a narrow one.

What I seek is a strong identity based on inclusion, not exclusion. This means that, while I cannot simply accept blindness, I must not reject it either. I must integrate it. I must try to relate blindness to sight, consciousness to unconsciousness, God to the devil, the life of humanity to the cosmos, the powers of creation to the powers of destruction. The stoic courageously tolerates these antitheses, but the one whose

Christian faith is in search of understanding must seek to go beyond these differences and to unite them.

Floating Away   *24 March 1985*

I am becoming rather abstract. I do not mean absent-minded, which is simply a matter of becoming very concrete about a particular thing. The absent-minded person is usually preoccupied because of concentration on something. My problem is abstraction. Everything is words and concepts, everything is speech. In addition, there are walls, and hedges, the feel of the pavement under my shoes, the vibration of my cane as I hold it, sometimes the feel of people's elbows or the fleeting touch of hands and fingers. That is more or less my world.

It is rich in human relationships. These relationships, however, have little background. They exist without a world. What is Birmingham? What is Selly Oak? What is the campus like these days? Has the ivy, which I used to watch year by year as it spread from either end of the Arts building, met in the centre yet? Is the University clock tower, Big Joe, different now that they have finished repointing it? I am told that the scaffolding is coming down. The conifers which were planted in University Square the year after I began my work here, and whose steady growth I watched with pleasure throughout the 1970s, how tall are they now? What are people wearing these days? One of my closest friends told me that he had gone almost entirely grey during the past five years. I had no idea.

This abstraction often gives me a sort of dreamy, floating feeling, as if I am drifting away from this life.

Still Looking   *25 March 1985*

I still have the feeling that I am looking. With the right eye, the one most recently blinded, I still have some sense of the macula, and I know how to turn my eyes from one side to another. I often do this automatically towards the place from which sounds come. So, in a sense, I still know how to look. Indeed, I still have a feeling that I am peering, gazing intently through the blackness, in case something should come into view.

I am not so sure if I am aware of doing this with the left eye, which has been totally blind for about thirty years. Sometimes I try the experiment of closing one eye and trying to imagine what I might be doing with the other. When both eyes are completely blind, however, it is extremely difficult to know whether I am really paying attention to this one rather than that one. I am helped a little by the fact that the right eye does still have some internal light sensation, although I cannot tell whether it is in the brain rather than the retina, and I do not know enough about it to know if either of these is more probable. From time to time, in the right eye, or with what I seem to be aware of when I pay attention to what I think is the right eye, a round area of fan-shaped pink or light orange light will appear. It will slowly roll around the 'visual field', the central area will then grow dark again, and the little display will then fade out towards the perimeter and disappear. It is quite interesting to 'watch' this.

Perhaps with a long-blinded eye one ceases to look, but with a recently blinded eye one is still looking. Perhaps the eye is switched off but the brain is still ready to receive some stimulation.

Sight and Darkness, Sound and Silence   *1 May 1985*

What corresponds visually to the difference between sound and silence? It cannot be the difference between seeing and shutting one's eyes, because you can always open your eyes and see again. It is within your power to grasp again the object of sense, but when there is silence, the ear has no power to grasp sound again. Even when your eyes are shut, you know that what you have seen is still there.

Does sound relate to silence as day relates to night? Surely not, for day and night are predictable, and even at night one sees a little. Is the relationship between sound and silence like that between seeing and being blind? Is blindness to sight as silence is to sound? This is clearly incorrect. Blindness is to sight as deafness is to sound. Blindness is an internal state. One knows that the external world is still there to be seen. One has merely lost the faculty of seeing it. In the case of silence, however, the external world, the world of sound, is not there any longer. It has gone into silence. In the case of silence one is still listening, but in the case of blindness, one can hardly be said to be still looking. You seldom look and see nothing, whereas you often listen but hear nothing, or very little. Whenever you look, the full range of your retina is always occupied with whatever there is to look at, but when you listen the full range of your hearing is not thus occupied with whatever there is to listen to. In total darkness, sight is useless. But in total silence, we would not say that the faculty of hearing was useless. It is just that there is nothing at the moment to hear.

It seems then that there is no exact visual parallel to the distinction between sound and silence. Sounds come and go in a way that sights do

145

not. Sounds have a gratuitous quality. One never possesses the sound, one never has it within one's power the way that one possesses the sight. The evil eye has power over the world, but nobody ever heard of an evil ear. The ability to close the eyes represents the power one has over things that are seen, the power to exclude. Hearing, however, is always receptive, whether to sound or to silence. You can look away, but you cannot listen away. You cannot turn the ear aside the way you can look aside. You can pretend that you don't hear, just as you can pretend that you don't see, but the ears cannot be averted.

Sound and silence come upon one from beyond. Sound is, however, experienced internally. Things seen are experienced objectively.

The sound/silence distinction is thus quite a powerful vehicle for the transcendent. It suggests that over which we have no power, which comes or does not come, which mysteriously starts and just as mysteriously finishes, to which we are always open but must remain attentive. This must be why it was always considered impious to look upon, but permissible to hear, God. Sound is transcendent.

God Is Heard but not Seen   *3 May 1985*

Perhaps a parallel to the experience of sound and silence would be suddenly entering a bank of fog when driving along the motorway. Beyond your power to affect it or predict it, the perceptual world is suddenly removed, only to emerge again on the other side. The difference is that fog is an obstruction to sight whereas silence is not an obstruction to hearing. Silence is an absence. Sound thus has absence built into it as its counterfoil, whereas sight does not. Sound is always bringing us into the presence of nothingness.

Perhaps this is why religions speak of not seeing God but seldom, if ever, of not hearing God. When we say that the Divine Being is invisible, we mean that we do not have power over it. To say that the Divine was inaudible, however, would be to claim that it had no power over us.

Gentle Death   *7 May 1985*

Yesterday I went out with my elder daughter for lunch. During the meal, I began to feel strangely remote. The waiters would not address any remark to me. Everything was said to Imogen, and I found it easiest to pass on my requests for service through her to the waiters. I should not have allowed that to happen, because it made me feel more remote. The fact that I was sitting not next to Imogen but opposite her also added to the feeling that she was not really there, and led me deeper into a sense of abstraction and isolation. One or two wisps of panic began to flicker through my brain, and when we arrived home, I felt completely exhausted.

I did not feel sleepy but had a desire to lie down under a blanket. I wanted to be warm and to forget. I felt extremely comfortable. I kept wondering what it would be like to lie down under a blanket of snow. I have read that people caught in snowstorms find that, if they give in to the temptation to lie down and rest, they often feel perfectly cosy, but they never wake up. I found myself wondering what it would be like if that were to happen to me now.

When I woke up after a couple of hours' sleep, the thought occurred to me that what I have been experiencing was not so much depression, since I felt rather happy, at least physically. My body felt relaxed. Had it been a sort of desire to die? Do people die in their sleep during such conditions? Can the psyche simply renounce life? Can the spirit simply not return? Can one commit suicide by mere desire?

Experiences like this have taught me that the deepest feelings go beyond feeling. One is numbed by the feeling; one does not experience the feeling. I recognize now, looking back, that I was in the grip of a profound melancholy due to the impoverishment of my rich relationship with a much-loved child, but at the time all I was conscious of was a desire to escape.

Intervals   19 May 1985

Any social exchange is punctuated by intervals. These become obvious when you listen to a tape-recorded conversation. You tend not to notice the intervals during the exchange itself. Between sighted people, there are accepted ways of filling these intervals. One gazes abstractly at the ceiling or glances at one's watch. For the blind person, the intervals are more difficult to handle because they become so much more ambiguous. For sighted people, when eye contact is removed, it is a signal of an interval. When eye contact is resumed, it is a signal that attention is regained and the exchange can continue. The blind person finds it more difficult to recognize a social interval. Has the person with whom one was talking simply got up and gone to the loo? Blind people also find it more difficult to time their own intervals, since they do not have the information provided by the facial expressions and the gestures of the other.

I try to handle these intervals partly through a lowered expectation.

I have to accept a certain impoverishment of the conversational relationship. If I continue to expect the same richness of moment-by-moment information about the other, I am bound to feel disappointed. The conversation which a blind person has takes place against a vastly reduced background of general information. Almost everything must be passed through the conversation itself. In the intervals, therefore, I must use inference and I must be patient. I must make guesses at what is going on, and I must recognize that, as a blind person, I will spend a great deal of my time sitting quietly, waiting for the interval to come to an end.

The danger is that I am waiting for the sighted person, only to discover that he or she has been waiting for me. We each sit there in expectant silence, because the normal cues for ending intervals are lacking.

These thoughts about intervals highlight for me certain characteristics of the blind person's relationship with others. These tend to be gratuitous, since it is more difficult to evoke them. They tend to be more fleeting, since they come and go. They tend also to be punctuated by these moments of waiting, of hope and of ignorance.

'You Know Me, Don't You?'   *20 May 1985*

I went to Staff House for lunch with a friend. As we passed through the doors into the foyer, I was in the middle of a group of people who greeted me with cries of, 'Now here's a surprise for you. Can you tell who this is?' Another voice broke through the noise saying, 'Do you recognize my voice, John?' I could not tell how many people there were, possibly four or five, maybe as many as seven or eight. Amongst the various voices, I recognized someone I knew and greeted him by name: Someone else was still asking me if I knew him, so I then turned towards him. With a laugh I said, 'No, I am ever so sorry, old chap. I'm afraid that I have no idea who you are. As far as I know, I have never met you before in my life. Now if you'll excuse me, I am going to the bar with my friend to get a drink.' I began to shoulder my way through them. This reply was met with howls of laughter, which was, I think, sympathetic towards me.

The voice continued, now more urgently, 'No, no. Come on John. You know me. You must know my voice, surely. We've been at conferences together.' Again, with a smile, I cheerfully replied, 'I really am sorry. It must be a terrible blow to your ego but I'm afraid that if we did happen to meet in the past, your impact upon me has been negligible.

I'm sure it must be very sad not to be recognized but there we are. You have left no trace upon my memory. Now, whoever you are, goodbye.' With this, I resumed my path towards the bar. Once again there were guffaws and hoots of laughter around the circle. At this, the man in question or somebody else grabbed me by the shoulder saying, 'It's blank blank.' I changed my manner, shook hands with him warmly and reminisced briefly about old times, saying how nice it was to meet him again.

In the quietness afterwards, I said to my companion, 'Do you think they meant to play all those silly games on me, or was it just spontaneous?' 'Oh no,' my friend replied, 'it was planned. I went through the door ahead of you, and I heard one of them say to the other, "Let's see if he can recognize your voice." '

This experience occurs from time to time. I am never quite sure what to make of it. People occasionally do this over the telephone to each other, but that is different. Each party on the end of a telephone is equal with respect to sight. I have various ways of trying to deal with it, and I think the method of cheerful scorn is quite successful. I do not want to hurt people's feelings, and to say boldly, 'No. I don't play silly games. If you want to talk to me you must tell me who you are', seems too harsh. What am I to do? Am I to stand there, feeling more and more foolish, suggesting name after name, while my interrogator with increasing impatience says, 'No. No. No. Try again'?

I have never had such a sharp sense of being the centre of a game of Blind Man's Buff as I did in the foyer of Staff House.

'He Turned into Banana Man' *7 June 1985*

When I put Lizzie to bed last night she was in rather a giggly mood. As I laid her down in the cot she said in a teasing voice, 'You can't see! You can't see!'

'Why can't I see?'

' 'Cos you're a blind man.'

'What's a blind man?' I asked.

Laughing, she replied, 'It's someone tall and strong and he turns into Banana Man.' This last expression was uttered with a shriek of delight.

Was she just fooling around? Does she know what blindness is or not? Is she associating blindness with other features of Daddy? I do pretend to be Banana Man when I am carrying her on my shoulders down the stairs. Or is she just telling me that I am a pompous old fool and both of us know perfectly well what a blind man is?

9

Waking Up Blind

Summer 1985

Amongst Blind People 17 *June 1985*

A few nights ago I attended the annual meeting of an association for the blind. This was the first time that I had been into a meeting attended by other blind people. Indeed, apart from occasional conversations with John Lorimer, the distinguished blind braillist who is on the staff of our Faculty, I have had almost no contact with other blind people, although it is now about five years since I lost my own sight.

It was curious and in a strange way rather comforting to find myself in a situation where the little habits which characterize the response of blind people to the world were accepted by a social group. The meeting began, for example, by everybody announcing who was present. This sometimes takes place in sighted groups when there is about to be a discussion, but I have never known it at the start of a business meeting. In the social exchange after the business meeting, there was a tremendous hubbub. People were simply shouting out the names of those they wanted to speak with, and in reply, you simply forced your way through the crowd towards whoever was shouting out your name.

I was told by two or three older blind men that the time of adjustment towards loss of sight grew longer in direct proportion to your age. For somebody of my age, I should consider five years quite a short time, and was assured that it would probably take me ten or fifteen years to make a full adjustment.

What Is It To Be with Someone?   *21 June 1985*

Marilyn happened to ask me if I had seen a certain colleague during the day. I knew that I had spoken with him, but had the curious sensation of not knowing whether I had been in his presence or not at the time. Was it face to face or was it on the telephone?

If I use the desk set and not the head set for a telephone call, the voice of my caller comes through so clearly in the room, while I am just sitting in my chair, that it is really quite similar to having the person with me. My colleague and I have a telephone link between our rooms, and often chat for a few minutes about a problem each day. I do not remember, however, that as a sighted person I ever had this strange hesitancy about whether I had been in the presence or not. This must be because a sighted person's memories of what was said are always associated with what was being seen at the time, so the words are either associated with the expression and posture of the speaker or with gazing at the traffic through the window as you made the telephone call. If this background information is stripped off, then the difference between the face-to-face situation and the telephone conversation is less. Of course, even for the blind person considerable differences remain, but the fact that I could experience this uncertainty shows that the difference has become rather fragile. If a slightly absent-minded person, at the end of a busy day, might wonder for a moment about the context in which he or she had met someone briefly, it is easy to see that as a blind person you will more often find yourself in that uncertainty. But the most absent-minded sighted person would not confuse speaking on the phone with being in the presence. The sighted person would only wonder whether it happened yesterday or today – 'it' would always be a meeting, or a telephone call.

This little moment of uncertainty tells us a great deal about blindness. As I paused, explaining to Marilyn that I was trying to work out whether we had been together or not, she sighed, and said, 'Oh dear! How strange! Even after all these years I still find it extremely difficult to realize what your experience of the world must be like.'

Lonely Parties   *23 June 1985*

You can see lots of things at once. Indeed, your visual field is made up of many hundreds, perhaps thousands, of tiny segments which are assembled into a totality. Your attention may be focused upon some particular item but the individual parts of what you see are not in direct competition. They are laid out alongside each other in space. In sound, however, one part of the acoustic field may actually obliterate the rest. The nearest visual parallel would be the experience of being dazzled. A bright shaft of light obliterates everything else. With sound, however, this happens much more readily. It is a characteristic of ordinary sounds, not just of exceptional sounds, although exceptional sounds certainly do wipe out other sounds.

When somebody turns the juke-box on in the coffee bar, the sound literally obliterates the voices of my friends. It is as if I was alone. They disappear. Only the juke-box exists. Its noise washes out all the rest of reality. It is as if you were painting, and you kept brushing over the water-colours with more and more colours, until all the distinctions vanished, and you were left with an even, grey smudge.

This must be why I find noisy parties, especially discos, so lonely. People have to tap me on the shoulder to attract my attention. It is like having headphones on and not being able to take them off.

What Is It To Be Somewhere?   *3 July 1985*

Marilyn asked me what I had done during the day, but for a moment I could not remember where I had been in the morning. I had been speaking with two colleagues, but where? It suddenly flashed upon me that I had spent the morning at Newman College.

This was not like the experience of a sighted but slightly absent-minded person who momentarily forgets what has been done during the day. I knew I had been somewhere, and had done particular things with certain people, but where? I could not put the conversations I had had into a context. There was no background, no features against which to identify the place. Normally, the memories of people you have spoken to during the day are stored in frames which include the background. You remember talking to the person and you remember that she was sitting in an armchair in front of a bookcase, or leaning against the window-sill through which the garden could be seen and so on. I knew that I had spoken with these people in some unusual context, because I could not associate my conversations with the usual sensations of my office chair and the feel of my elbows on the desk.

It was this strange sense of blankness which was so disconcerting. It reminds me of the incident the other day when I could not, for a moment, remember whether I had been in the presence of Michael when I had a conversation with him. What someone says is normally associated with the look on her face as she says it, and with her posture and what she is wearing. The body in turn is situated against its own background.

So I was at Newman College. But what does it mean to me? What does the concrete, physical presence of the College buildings mean? I have taught with these people in what they told me was 'Newman College'. It could have been anywhere else. We walked up and down stairs and along corridors. We sat down in what was described as the Principal's office. All this, however, could have been anywhere. The blind person's experience of institutions is rather abstract.

Touch Is Beautiful   *4 July 1985*

It is now many months since I began to appreciate the illumination and sense of real knowledge which comes through touch. In more recent weeks, I am beginning to experience not only this real knowledge through touch but also the pleasure of it. The other day I was at the home of a friend whose wife collects model owls. He put into my hand a little stone owl about five inches high. It was squat and beautifully rough. The weight of it in my hand was satisfying. There was a carved, wooden owl from Africa. I admired the simplicity of the details, the warmth and smoothness of the wood, the way that the whole object could be contained within the hand.

I am developing the art of gazing with my hands. I like to hold and rehold and go on holding a beautiful object, absorbing every aspect of it. In a multi-cultural exhibition the other day, I was allowed to handle a string of beads, smooth and polished, and a South American water jar made from earthenware. There was a lovely, scraping sound when one rotated the lid of the jar, and thousands of tiny, tinkling, hollow echoes were made when the full, round belly of the jar was touched with the fingernails.

I am beginning to enjoy the different textures of materials. One of my teacher friends is using a heavy, velvet bag to conceal an object from her children. They have to feel it through the bag. I love the way the fibres wiggle as your hands pass over the bag, this way and that. There is a delightful contrast with the smooth clean sharpness of the metal bracelet in the bag.

I am surprised that it should have taken approximately five years to begin to appreciate experiences of this kind. Weight, texture and shape, temperature and the sounds things make, these are what I look for now.

'You're Blind and I'm not Very Strong' *14 July 1985*

During breakfast the other day I called out to Marilyn, who was struggling with a million other things, 'Have you made the tea yet, darling?'

'Yes,' she called back from the kitchen. 'It's on the table in front of you.'

Lizzie interjected, 'Why did you ask Mummy for the tea?'

Thomas said, 'It's because he had to ask Mummy.'

Lizzie added, 'It's because you can't see and I can see.'

I thought this was a good example of Lizzie's increasing ability to interpret my otherwise extraordinary behaviour.

As I was standing in the front porch with Thomas, looking down the steps towards the car which was parked in the road, Thomas asked, 'Why don't we park the car in the house?'

'We'd have a job getting up the steps,' I replied.

'Why?' he asked.

'Have you ever tried to lift it?'

'No.'

'Well, it's pretty heavy,' I said. 'Anyway,' I continued, 'we might try it. You could take one end and I could take the other.'

'Well', he said in a serious but rather doubtful tone, 'it would be difficult. You're blind and I'm not very strong.'

'We could get Lizzie,' I suggested.

'She's not very strong either,' he mused.

'What about Mummy?' I asked.

'Well . . .' he sounded most uncertain.

'Let's face it,' I said briskly, 'the whole family's not very strong.'

He did not seem inclined to pursue this any further, and changed the subject.

'Jesus Will Heal You'   *15 July 1985*

On Friday I went to New Street Station to meet a friend. As I moved across the concourse, I was approached by a chatty Irishman who escorted me to a suitable position where I would be seen by my guest as she came through the barriers. Having put me into position, he asked if I would mind some personal questions. I told him to go ahead, and he asked me if it was true that I was blind. I confirmed this, and without further ado, he declared, 'Jesus will heal you.' I responded to this in vigorous religious terms, assuring him that he need have no anxiety. Jesus had already given me his presence and his guidance and although my outward sight was decayed I hoped that my inward vision was getting stronger every day. Moving the discussion to his life, I found out that he was a Pentecostalist, and we talked about this for some time.

The arrival of my train was announced, and my friend told me that he had a young daughter injured in a hit-and-run road accident. She was in hospital, he had to go and see her, but he had no money to give her a gift. Would I be kind enough to help him to buy a bunch of grapes for her? I gave him the required sum and we parted with mutual praising of the Lord.

Does Blindness Make You More Efficient? 16 July 1985

Marilyn told me that a sensitive friend had asked her whether it was my blindness which, through helping me to concentrate more, had been responsible for the creativity which she thinks I have shown during the last six months or so.

There may be something in this. Blindness is like a huge vacuum cleaner which comes down upon your life, sucking almost everything away. Your past memories, your interests, your perception of time and how you will spend it, place itself, even the world, everything is sucked out. Your consciousness is evacuated, and you are left to reconstruct it, including a new sense of time, a new realization of the body in space and so on. In that situation, there is likely to be a drastic revision of priorities. As for my own so-called creativity during these months, for what it is worth, it must be remembered that from 1968 until about 1983 I was completely occupied by my teaching and supervising duties with students, and my university committee work. No less important than the onset of my blindness is the fact that since about 1983, through the natural process of not seeking re-election, I have given up most of my university committees including Court, Council, Senate, Academic Executive, Faculty Board, Education General Purposes Committee and lots of lesser committees. It is quite possible that, had I been relieved of those duties and retained my sight, I would have been just as creative in research and publications as perhaps I have been these last few months.

It is also true that I spent the first three or four years after my loss of sight in getting my university teaching work together. It was not really until the beginning of the 1984/5 academic year that I began to feel confident. The time which I had spent on making notes on cassette so I could resource my teaching work could now be diverted into more original writing.

Taking all of these factors into account, I still think there is something purging about blindness. One must re-create one's life or be destroyed. I was fortunate in that I had such a strong central core to my life. I had a job, a secure family life, an institution which accepted me and helped me, and multitudes of friends.

Movements   *19 July 1985*

I can tell when other things are moving by the sounds they make. Cars swish past, feet patter along, leaves rustle, but a silent nature is immobile. So it is that, for me, the clouds do not move, the world outside the car window or the window of the train is not moving. The countryside makes no noise as the train passes through it. The hills and fields are silent.

If the movements of other bodies are revealed by sound, the movements of my own body are revealed by the fact that it is being made to vibrate, or I feel the sway of the carriage as we round the bend at high speed. I am held back in my seat as we accelerate, and thrust forward as we slow down.

This means, however, that the knowledge I have of my own body's movements and of the movements of other things is not symmetrical. The cues are provided by external sound and internal sensation. This is not the case for sighted people, who can tell whether other things are moving and whether they themselves are moving by the same faculty of sight. You know when the train starts by looking out of the window. You tell it, as a sighted person, by seeing a changing relationship between your body and the world. The different ways in which the blind person experiences motion indicate that the normal relationship between the body and the world has been severed.

Walking   *21 July 1985*

When she is out walking, the sighted person sees a world within potential reach. She knows that by performing a certain amount of work (i.e. walking) she will turn that potential into an actual reach. A measured, predictable quantity of walking will bring the anticipated object closer. The walking of the sighted person thus has purpose. Her purpose is to get to a certain point which she already envisages. This is illustrated by the fact that sighted people tend to become discouraged when objects towards which they are walking, like a distant line of hills, do not seem to be any nearer after putting in a lot of work.

The problem of walking for the blind person is that you have no world of potential reach, but only a zone of actual reach, made up by the feeling of your feet on the ground. You do not know if a bend in the road is in sight, or if there is a range of hills ahead. The blind person thus lacks an incentive to form a purposeful action which would turn something grasped potentially into something realized actually.

The result is that the blind person, when walking, becomes mainly conscious of his or her own body. There are movements up and down, steps one after the other. There is, of course, a pleasure in feeling the wind in one's face, the sound of the birds, and the smells, but all this could be experienced if one was stationary. If the blind person is walking along a familiar route, then it is better. Through memory, I know that a certain amount of work will bring me to a particular point, where we sat on the fallen log, for example, where there is a bridge and we will be able to lean on it and listen to the river. Because the route is familiar, the blind walker can estimate how much work it will take to get to that point. A new route, without information, can easily become rather meaningless.

When I am walking along the city streets, along a strange route, escorted by a friend, I tend to ask frequently such questions as, 'Can you see it yet? Is it a long block? How far do you think it will be now?' I seem to need to set my body to reach certain goals in a walk which otherwise will become a weary plod. There is so little progress; the things now passing were not far off a moment ago. It is easy for a blind person to have the feeling that a lot of work is being done but little progress is being made.

Only if the route is punctuated by various textures of the pavement, the smell of a bakery or the sounds of a street musician, is there a feeling of having crossed an area, drawn near to things and gone past them.

Is There Shape without Colour?   *29 July 1985*

A philosophical friend remarked that there can be no shape without colour and no colour without shape. Colour and shape are absolutely inseparable. Nevertheless, they are easily distinguishable.

This is surely false. Shape and colour are entirely separable. I, for example, continually experience shapes that have no colours at all. It would be more accurate to say that shapes and textures are inseparable but distinguishable. A sighted person might object that clouds have shapes but no textures, and what about the sky itself? My reply is that 'clouds' and 'sky' are mere words which have no place in my own experience of life. I do not dispute what you say because I cannot. I can only report that in my own experience there are never shapes without textures nor textures without shapes. There are things which have neither shape nor texture, like wind and water. I notice in passing that the relationship which a sighted person experiences between things which have shape and colour and those which do not is not the same as the relationship which the blind person experiences between things which have shape and texture and those which do not. These latter, for the blind person, remain tangible, although without shape or texture. One feels the wind; one feels water. For a sighted person, on the other hand, that which has neither shape nor colour is simply invisible. Shape and colour exhaust the visual sense without remainder. Shape and texture do not exhaust the tactile sense without remainder, because one also has the wet/dry sensation, the hot/cool sensation and the light/heavy sense of pressure. All of these can be appreciated by touch independently of texture.

What the philosophers should say is that the *sight* of shapes is always inseparable from its colours, or that visually, shape and colour are inseparable yet distinguishable. Unconsciously, the shadow of the sighted person's consciousness falls upon the page.

Waking Up and Going Blind   *8 August 1985*

A few minutes ago I drifted off to sleep in my armchair on this Saturday afternoon in the office. I dreamed that my colleague, Michael, knocked on my door to tell me that he was finishing work and going home. He closed the door and left. Then an unbelievable thing happened. My room was flooded with light. With incredulity, I gazed at the walls and saw the rows of books, filing cases and labelled boxes, all in bright colours and standing out clearly and neatly with an amazing simplicity of line, form and colour. I couldn't believe my eyes. The whole room was aglow with objects. I daren't blink in case it should disappear. I got to my feet, terrified lest the change of position should suddenly make me realize this was a dream. I staggered to the door, thinking as I stretched out my hand to grasp the door handle how remarkable it was to be able to do that. Reaching the door, I looked back into the room, seeing it now from a different perspective. There was the desk with all the things on it, as fresh and bright and distinct as if it was the very day of creation. Out into the corridor I stumbled, crying out, 'Mike! Mike!' My voice couldn't get out. It was choked. I realized that, although I was struggling to scream, what was coming out was no more than a whisper. In the corridor it was gloomy, but I could still see. As I hurried towards the lift, I was moving my hands side to side as if I was waving my stick. I don't think I had actually taken the stick off its hook beside the door. The thought crossed my mind, 'There's no need for me to do that now.

Now that I can see. But how hard it will be to throw off that habit of moving my hand from side to side.' I was wondering what on earth could have happened to my eyes to have brought this thing about.

Up the steps now I dashed, and around the foyer to the lift. Michael, with his wife and family, were just getting in. No, indeed, they had entered, and the doors were closing. I hurried forward. The doors of the lift closed. I felt now as if I was about to faint. I hammered on the metal doors as I saw, through the little window, the lift going down. Again I cried out, but all that came was a muffled hoarse whisper. The lift disappeared, and as I stood there, the vision began to fade. The distinction between the blue, metal doors and the brown jambs on either side began to blur, it began to melt and disappear. Mists and darkness came flooding in. I was back in consciousness. And there I was, in my chair, and I realized with a shock that it had been a dream.

Within this dream there is a consciousness of being blind, since I am a blind person who, in the dream, regains sight and loses it again. The curious feature is that, although the regaining of sight is part of the dreamed story, the loss of sight is not, so to speak, something I dream about. In the dream, I do not dream that I lose my sight. What happens is simply that I wake up. As I stand beside the closed lift doors, I do not dream that I go blind. All that happens is that the vision is swept away by returning consciousness. The dream stops because I wake up. The fear, in the dream, of moving lest I should lose my sight is the same as the fear that I should move in my chair, and disturb the dream and so wake up too soon.

The simultaneity of the experience of waking up and of going blind impresses me. I stood beside the lift doors. The little lighted panel was going down, with a fleeting glimpse of Michael and his family. Then it began to fade away, as with a moment of panic and despair I realized that I was both waking up and losing my sight. I opened my eyes and my mind grew dark. Every time I return to consciousness I lose my sight again.

I do not remember any dream which has left me with such a sharp sense of reality-shock as this one. This is partly due to the continuity between the dream and the actual circumstances in which I fell asleep. It was all so natural, so plausible, there was such a smooth continuity of events. The reality of it all was completely overwhelming, and the movement back from the dream-reality to the actual reality left my mind numbed, as with a blow. It was not merely the realization again that I am blind, but the strange sense of passing from one reality to another, as if my mind had become derailed. There had been a sort of reality clock. Everything was swimming around me. The vivid distinctness of perceived objects was now exchanged for the feel of my body and clothes on the armchair, the smooth edge of the desk at which I was sitting, the knowledge that all I knew was confined within the reach of my fingers. Everything else had gone again. I felt deceived, momentarily uncertain as to whether this might also be an interlude in the dream, and if I sat very still it also might fade away.

Body-image and Body-awareness   *9 August 1985*

The place of the image of my own body is being gradually taken by a sort of awareness of the bodily field. Internal awareness of the size, relations and position of one's body seems to gradually take the place of the external images of bodily posture.

Sometimes during a meeting, when I was gradually losing my sight, I would look down at my knees, tracing the line of the trousers down to my shoes and up again, and I would think how strange it would be not to know what my own body was doing by looking at it. When this is replaced by internal or subjective bodily awareness, although pleasure remains, and there can be a sense of balance, of well-being, one loses the sense of beauty and grace. In my own case, that is certainly no great loss, but I wonder how other blind people feel about this. There is a pleasure in seeing the symmetry of the body. I have two arms. I feel the clothing on each arm, I can wave each hand in the air, I can hold my head with both hands. This does give a certain pleasurable feeling of symmetry, but it is no longer aesthetic, as is the visual image of the gracious proportion of the human body.

Memorizing Milton   *10 August 1985*

I began to memorize the first book of *Paradise Lost*. I am now up to line 350. This has been a very good experience and has become part of my answer to the persistent problem: what fills the consciousness of the blind person?

A blind person spends a lot of time just waiting for sighted people. Now, I have something to think about, something to work at while I am waiting. I know my route to work so well that, except for the Bristol Road crossing and a short section at the end where I have to actually count the steps between a number of lampposts, I can recite Milton to myself as I go along. It is also a comfort to know that I have this resource, I can enjoy this majestic language at will. I don't have to have the cassette player. I don't have to worry about braille. I can read it any time I like simply by thinking about it.

I am also enjoying a rapport with Milton himself. I wonder how he managed it. Did he memorize what he had written each day? I also find that many of the familiar passages take on new meaning when I think of them as a communication from a blind person to me.

Before you begin to memorize the next section, you wonder how you will do it. In advance, it often seems very complex. In retrospect, after memorization, it appears to be strangely foreshortened and is now a mere interlude before the next part. I suppose to those heroic minds who have memorized all twelve books, the whole of Books One and Two seem nothing but a prelude. Here is a clue about how to tackle such impossible tasks. Mountains become hills by climbing them.

The Fifth Anniversary: Stages of the Journey   *11 August 1985*

In commemoration of the fifth anniversary of my final eye operation, I want to set out the stages through which this journey has passed.

First, there was a period of hope which lasted for a year or eighteen months. It was brought to an end by the deterioration of sight during the summer of 1981, although even as late as the summer of 1982, when I was still seeing a few lights, colours and shapes, I could not resist occasional flickers of hope.

Secondly, there was a period of business in overcoming the problems. This began about the summer of 1981, when visual work became impossible, and lasted until about the summer of 1984. It was not until Easter of 1985 that I began to have a feeling that I did not need any more equipment. The main drive to create a workable office system took place during 1982 and 1983. During this time, blindness was a challenge.

The third stage began some time in 1983, possibly late in the year, and lasted for about a year. This was the time when I passed through despair. These were the years during which my sleep was punctuated by terrible dreams, and my waking life was oppressed by the awareness of being carried irresistibly deeper and deeper into blindness.

The fourth and current period has begun since the autumn of 1984, that is since the recovery from my visit to Australia, during which time blindness had engulfed me. I began writing my book on adult religious education in October of 1984 and concluded it in March 1985.

For most of the time now my brain no longer hurts with the pain of blindness. There has been a strange change in the state or the kind of activity in my brain. It seems to have turned in upon itself to find inner resources. Being denied the stimulus of much of the outside world, it has had to sort out its own functions and priorities. I now feel clearer, more excited and more adventurous intellectually than ever before in my life. I find myself connecting more, remembering more, making more links in my mind between the various things I have read and had to learn over the years. Sometimes I come home in the evening and feel that my mind is almost bursting with new ideas and new horizons.

I continue to find a deep need for that kind of sustenance. Even a single day without study, away from the possibility of learning something new, can precipitate a new sense of urgency and suffering. I still feel like a person on a kidney machine, but increasingly like a person who has managed to survive.

10

Lost Children

Autumn 1985

Entering a Birthday World   *1 September 1985*

During the party to celebrate Thomas's fifth birthday, a child came over and sat on my knee. At first, I thought it was Lizzie, but as time went by, I became more and more uncertain. I reached the point where the only way I could be sure was by asking, 'What's your name?' I shrank from this in case it really was Lizzie. She would then know that I had not recognized her. This was rather a puzzling and even distressing situation.

When a child opens a birthday present, everybody admires it. It is silly for me to join in these cries of admiration, because everybody would know that I was pretending. I tried sitting Thomas on my knee so I could get some idea of what the object was, but the trouble is that my hands get in his way, and without touching I do not know. In any case, it is seldom that after a moment or two of touching you can give a gasp of surprise and delight. Knowledge by touch takes time. In any case, the child will not stay on your knee, but keeps running off to get more presents and to show them to other admirers. It is impossible not to experience a creepy sense of remoteness at such a time.

After the children had all gone, Thomas came running up to me with a new set of mathematical puzzles in the form of playing cards. He wanted me to do this with him. I tried to explain that I could not help him much, and he pulled from his pocket another puzzle. This is set into a clear plastic case, and is one of those puzzles where you have to roll little silver balls around until they come to rest in little holes. With a sick feeling, I tried to explain that this one was even more difficult for me. Undeterred, he produced a board game. We opened it. With a sinking heart, I realized that all of the counters were exactly the same. They must have been different colours but they all felt alike. The board was completely smooth. I suggested that Mummy would help him later. I tried to enthuse over all these presents, but it was hard work. I fell asleep that night like a worn-out ghost.

In the morning I took a new initiative. When Thomas ran in at about seven o'clock, I told him to go and get all the things he had been given for his birthday, bring them all up and spread them out on the bed, and I would go through every one of them with him. He was delighted and this worked very well. Laying things out on the bed, one by one, in the quietness, I was able to get his description of every toy or game while I had time to explore each item carefully, discovering all I could about it, and working out whether there would be any way that I could use it with him. Without the social pressure to express premature admiration, I could enjoy this very much. To some extent, I had entered his birthday world.

Leading Daddy   6 September 1985

Two or three times this week I have walked with Thomas to his school. Perhaps I should say that he has walked with me, for he is getting quite good at guiding me. He walks nearest the road holding my hand, while I use the cane to keep me clear of the front fences. He is old enough not to walk out on to the road, and in any case, provided that I keep close to the walls and fences, I can hold him well inside the footpath. He has learned how to give my hand a little tug towards him when he sees that I am about to walk into a hedge or gatepost. He is, however, unreliable about this, and if I am not alert with the cane, I will sometimes walk smack bang into a post because he is watching something else.

I have also worked out a very satisfactory way of saying goodbye to him at the school gate. As he runs off through the playground, he calls back to me, ' 'bye'. I respond by calling out ' 'bye' and we exchange these calls, getting fainter and fainter as he runs further and further away, until at last his calls disappear into the general background noise of the school yard. As I am turning round to go, having waved as hard as I can, I hear one final, faint little call, ' 'bye'. This game avoids the abrupt and disconcerting disappearance which is the usual experience of a blind person saying goodbye to someone. The echoing calls provide an intermediate stage for a gradual disappearance, and this is almost as good as seeing each other wave.

Lizzie is also interested in leading me, and there is a certain good-natured competition entering into this. Often I have Thomas on one hand and Lizzie on the other. I enjoy this very much, but it makes it difficult to use the cane. I am all right provided they don't decide to walk one on each side of a post. Daddy in the middle collects it. Lizzie is very proud of her skill, and calls out to Marilyn, 'Look! I am leading Daddy. I'm showing Daddy. I'm showing him.'

Ludo   *7 September 1985*

Blind person's Ludo has been a great asset. I played happily with the children all day until four in the afternoon. After the Ludo, we played 'Reversi' on a board also designed for blind people, but just as good for the sighted, and then Thomas and I listened to some old Goon Show cassettes, with satisfactory results all round. We then played a card game called 'Jumble Sales' and several other board games.

Even when we are not playing a game which is adapted for blind people, I do not seem to find it as upsetting as once I did. I seem to be more content just to sit there, and be told what to do, to shake the dice, to keep up an enthusiastic commentary, which the children seem to find a perfectly adequate kind of participation. The truth is that often I have little or no idea what the rules of the game are, and sometimes I am not even sure which game we are playing.

Gabriel   *8 September 1985*

Gabriel is less than a month old, and I am enjoying his company very much. I love the smell of him, and the way he breathes in rapid little pants when I call his name. I love to feel the way his head twists around when Marilyn enters the room, and the way he turns back to look at me. I love the feel of him when he goes to sleep in my arms, the change in the sound and pattern of his breathing. I love holding his tiny hands and putting my own hand on the warmth of his head. I like to feel whether his hair is growing and I like feeling his little nose. I like holding one of his feet and I like the feel of his whole body as I hold him over one shoulder. All of these things are very much less spoiled by the lack of sight than was the case with either Thomas or Lizzie. I have some pangs of regret when somebody remarks, 'He's smiling at you' or, 'What a bright, alert baby you've got there!' Provided that such thoughts do not come to the front of my mind too much, I find that I am getting much more genuine and immediate pleasure from this little baby. He is well named.

Lost Children   *3 October 1985*

Last night I dreamed that the family and I were shopping in a supermarket or department store which was built over a cliff. A huge wave crashed down on the store, separating us all. I rushed back to the flooded shop; looking for the children. There was debris everywhere, flooded bales of cloth, merchandise and dead bodies. Marilyn, Gabriel and Imogen were safe at the top end of the shop. It was Thomas and Elizabeth who were missing. They had been down, below the level to which the water had come. I searched for them everywhere, in growing despair, finding nothing. I came back and told Marilyn there was no sign of them. We were all full of grief, and continued to search everywhere, but it was hopeless. They had simply disappeared. We erected a small plaque in memory of them. There was a lot of discussion about what we should say. Should we simply say that the sea took them? Now I am down on the cliff-edge myself, still searching for them. The cliff is very rugged and steep, and is composed of masses of thin layers of slate or shale. This seems to have been loosened by the impact of the wave, and as I clamber around the edge, hanging out over the wild sea, huge pieces of shale slide off under the pressure of my feet or fingertips and crash down. I am scrabbling around for my toe-hold, wondering if the entire cliff face will crumble and collapse. As I stretch out, trying to obtain a grip, huge slabs of rock slide away with a rush of rubble and debris. Other people are clambering around, higher up. At last, somehow, I manage to scramble up to where the cliff face seems less affected by the wave and storm and to be reasonably solid. So I manage to escape, but still there is no sign of Thomas or Lizzie.

This dream seemed to be immensely long. I awoke from it very gradually. Indeed, I am not quite sure at what point the dream ended and the nightmarish fantasy began. There was no sharp sense of division between the dream and reality, and the dream flooded my waking consciousness with a sense of dread.

Earlier in the summer, a group of school children had been swept off the rocks in Cornwall. This incident made a deep impression upon me, as did a dream which one of my colleagues recently told me, in which her children had been drowned on the rocks. The dream is basically about the loss in family relationships which blindness causes. Thomas and Lizzie, who are just learning to understand blindness, are drowned beneath it. Imogen was born before the shock and Gabriel after it. The dream also suggests that fragments of my old life, my conscious, sighted life, are sliding and crashing down all around me into the all-engulfing world of blindness.

Wild Geese   13 October 1985

We went to a party to celebrate the ordination of one of our ministers. A singing group called 'Wild Geese' had come down from Glasgow to take part. Twice during the evening, this choir of a dozen or so young people gathered on the stairs of the house and sang African liberation songs. I stood very close to them with Thomas on my shoulders. He was beating to the music, and clapping his hands. The music was so rich and exciting. I felt exhilarated and blessed. Over the noise of the clapping and singing, Thomas shouted into my ear, 'What are they singing about?'

'They're singing about freedom,' I replied. He laughed with delight and so did I.

Later in the evening somebody said to me, 'John, you might like to know that all those young people look so radiant, their faces are smiling, and they are dressed in such bright colours! Some are in red and orange, others are dressed like harlequins with alternate squares of coloured cloth, and they all look so happy!'

I was glad to have this information, because I had pictured them as dressed in tartans with white blouses and lots of lace. I do not suppose I will ever be able to avoid forming some mental image or other, and since this should always be as realistic as possible, I am always glad to have more information.

What moved me, however, was the sound. I do not think that my pleasure at the noise of the singing could have been increased by sight, or by a description at some earlier point of what I would have seen. I do not believe that my feeling of blessedness lacked anything because the visual element was absent. I felt slightly upset that some people might think that there would be some deficiency in my enjoyment of all this.

As one goes deeper and deeper into blindness the things which once were taken for granted, and which were then mourned over as they disappeared, and for which one tried in various ways to find compensation, in the end cease to matter. Somehow, it no longer seems important what people look like, or what cities look like. One cannot check at first hand the accuracy of these reports, they lose personal meaning and are relegated to the edge of awareness. They become irrelevant in the conduct of one's life. One begins to live by other interests, other values. One begins to take up residence in another world.

I think that I may be beginning to understand what blindness is like.

Bells   *28 October 1985*

Marilyn and I were invited to the wedding of a friend. This took place in a village church, which had been chosen because of its picturesque qualities. As we were leaving the building, the mother of the groom said to me, 'What a pity that you can't see the church! It really is so lovely. It's such a sweet little church. It is a pity you can't see it.' I smiled vaguely and we walked outside. The bells were ringing. Someone else approached us, remarking on how beautiful the ceremony was. Again, the groom's mother said, 'But what a pity it was John couldn't see the church!' After the photographs had been taken, with the pretty little church as a background, I found myself again with the groom's mother, this time with Marilyn. For the third time, the same observations were made. 'What a pity John couldn't see the pretty church.' Marilyn and I laughed it off and changed the subject.

This makes me reflect on the psychology of sighted people. Our benign hostess, who had chosen the church because it looked so pretty, felt slightly frustrated because she was unable to be a good hostess as far as I was concerned. The whole point of having the ceremony was lost on me. The site had been chosen to give visual pleasure. I could not derive such pleasure. Therefore, it was a pity. The pity, to be quite accurate about it, was not so much that I couldn't see it, but that all the trouble had been gone through, as far as I was concerned, for nothing. It was a pity to do all that work and make all those plans for nothing.

This raises the additional reflection that I am not recruitable by sighted people. I am not entertainable, in the way sighted people know entertainment. It is impossible to draw me into the general admiration of what has been laid on to be admired. This becomes a pity.

When I am in such a place, I am not preoccupied by the thought that there are things I cannot see. My attention and my emotions are occupied by what actually presses in upon me.

In this case, it was the bells. I could have stood there, listening to those bells, for a long time. The air was full of the vibrations. My head seemed to be ringing. The ground seemed to be trembling, and the very air was heavy and springy with the reverberations. I tried to count how many different patterns they were ringing, and, without success, to work out how many bells must be in the tower. I thought that I really must become more expert in this lovely thing. I tried to describe the qualities of the sound to myself, mentally comparing it with other bells I had recently heard. Again and again, the descending peals chimed out, over the babble of conversation, cutting up the cool autumnal air, weighting everything with a strange, solemn expectancy. I was flooded with joy, and repeated again and again in my heart, 'Yes, I hear you, dear bells, I hear you.'

I might not have reacted in this way had I already known the place. When I return to a familiar place, like the chapel of King's College in Cambridge, I am often full of a very strong sense of loss. In a new place, however, I usually don't bother much about what it might look like. I just write that off as unavailable, and concentrate upon those parts of it which can get through to me. Indeed, it disturbs me to be given information about the appearance of something, unless I specifically ask for it. Often, I do ask, because I am curious. There may be certain details I want to know. There is no value in ignorance. Sometimes, on those occasions, I will interrogate a sighted friend in some detail. The initiative, however, has to be mine.

I do not know whether the sighted people even noticed the bells. At best they could have been only an extra item of atmosphere, added to the autumn leaves and the Norman tower as the bridal party gathered in their beautiful clothes. To me, the very air I was breathing was bell-shaped.

Heat   *15 November 1985*

Sitting at the dining-room table the other day I became aware of heat falling upon my face. I traced it to its source by moving my face and hands around, and finally located it in the light bulb which was hanging from the ceiling above me. I cannot remember ever having had this experience before. Since then, I have been paying attention, and I find that I can often tell whether the light in a room is on or not just by standing beneath it with my face uplifted. I am also much more aware of rays of sunlight falling across my face. Indeed, the whole of my skin seems to have become much more sensitive to changes of pressure and temperature, to wind and sun.

A Put Down?   *18 November 1985*

The other day, I attended a meeting of about twenty colleagues. The speaker seemed to be a particularly kind-hearted person, very sensitive to the needs of a blind person. She drew me into her talk by offering special explanations of things. As she held something up, she would remark, 'Now you wouldn't know this, John, but so and so and so and so' or 'John, you might like to know that this coloured so and so . . .' or 'For your benefit, John, I'm holding up a . . .' or 'It grieves me more than I can say that you can't see this beautiful flag, John, but it's a so and so and a so and so.' I nodded politely to all this, trying to look intelligent and appreciative.

No doubt, people who value me regret that they cannot recruit me to admire the things they admire. Still, facts must be faced. Since I am not recruitable, it seems pointless to draw attention to it in this way, with lamentations and expostulations of grief. This has the effect of making me feel an outsider. Just as I am getting interested in what is being said, there comes the stabbing reminder, again and again; you are outside this; you are not one of us. Is it possible that sometimes this is intended? Is it possible that this could be a sighted person's defence against the power of my powerlessness? How do you successfully put down a blind person?

From Accident to Meaning   *22 December 1985*

Was there a meaning in it? Was I meant to go blind? People often ask me questions like these.

My blindness was the result of thousands of tiny accidental happenings. These were not a 'path' and I was not being led along it towards blindness. Looking back, I can see the chain of events, and it looks a bit like a path, but any trackless waste is laid out with paths once it has been crossed. When you look ahead, there is no path but only an almost infinite number of possibilities.

The word 'providence' means 'looking ahead' and traditionally refers to the idea that God leads you along a path. I believe that we should call this doctrine retrovidence, or looking back, because it is only as we look back that the fortuitous is endowed with meaning. Meaning is conferred after the event. This is why the question 'why did this happen?' is rather a misleading one. It happened because I happened to be born in the twentieth century and not in the nineteenth. If I had been born a hundred years ago, no doubt I should have lost my sight at a much earlier age; if I had been born a century from now, no doubt my sight would have been saved. In other words, I could describe a thousand little ifs and buts which could give some account of how it was that this event took place in the life of this individual. But if by 'why' one is asking about the overall purpose, as if blindness itself was my fate, I do not believe it.

Each of the events which preceded the big event was fortuitous, and the entire sequence had no more probability within it than was accumulated as each accidental event prepared the way, more or less, for the next.

Faith is a creative act. It is through faith that we transform the accidental events of our lives into the signs of our destiny. Happiness is fortuitous but meaning is conferred when chance is transfigured through a rebirth of images.

This, however, is not an achievement, or at least it is not experienced as the result of effort. Images have their own energy, and the meaningful life is experienced as those images restructure the accidental content of life. The most important thing in life is not happiness but meaning. Happiness is the product of chains of accident which tend towards our well-being. Blindness does not make me happy. I did not choose it, nor was it inflicted upon me. Nevertheless, as an accidental event it could become meaningful. Retrovidence is a visionary gift.

11

The Gift

Winter 1985/Spring 1986

'Why Doesn't God Help You?'   *28 December 1985*

Last Friday night, as I was putting him to bed, Thomas launched into a long and detailed discussion about my blindness. 'Will you always be blind?' was his opening thought.

'Yes, always.'

'Even on the Last Day?'

'Yes.'

'When did it happen? Was it when I was a little boy or a baby?'

'No. It was before you were born, just before you were born.'

'What was it like? Did you have one good eye that you could see with and one bad eye that you couldn't see with and then your good eye got worse? Or did you have two good eyes or what?'

'I had one good eye that I could see with but it gradually got worse.'

'Couldn't the doctors stop it?'

'The doctors tried.'

'What was wrong with it? Why did it get worse?'

I then explained to him about detached retina. I told him about the retina of the eye, what it is and a little bit about how it works. I described how the retina may become elevated from the back of the eye or torn and what effect this has.

'Why does it tear? What makes it come off? Can't they put it back on?'

I described the many operations I had had, and told him something of the techniques used in trying to replace the retina and prevent further

172

elevations. I described how gradually it had got worse and worse, and how other complications had set in.

'Couldn't they do any more in the end? What did they say?'

'Well,' I told him, 'they just said "We're very sorry, Mr Hull, we are afraid that there isn't much more we can do now." '

'That was bad luck,' he said.

I agreed.

'Why doesn't God help you?'

'God does help me, in lots of ways.'

'How?'

'Well, he makes me strong. He gives me courage.'

'But he doesn't help you to get your eyes back.'

'No, but he does help me with lots of other things, and he has helped me with lots of other things.'

At this point I felt that he had enough to think about, and so did I; I went off to have my supper and he went to sleep. This discussion must be put into the context of Thomas's current theology, which is a theology of divine power, based upon what He-man and Superman can do. God is seen as the perfection of He-man and Superman, rolled into one but stronger than them both. The film *Superman* had been on the television only the previous day and the children had watched it with great interest. Superman is a deliverer, a saviour and a liberator who shows amazing strength and resourcefulness on behalf of his friends and fellow-countrymen. By contrast, the outcome of having God as one's ally seems disappointing.

I think that Thomas needs time, as I do, to come to God in his own way. The image he has of the Divine now does have the power to arouse wonder and awe, and is suitable for a five-year-old boy. Ultimately, however, for a Christian a theology of power needs to come to grips with a theology of weakness and of the cross. Power is easy to visualize, powerlessness is much more difficult. It takes great strength to have a theology of weakness, but one cannot expect a young child to grasp that. I am not sure that I grasp it myself.

I was, however, impressed by the nature of his questioning, the interest and the details of the surgery and the ophthalmology, and what I had felt about it. I was struck by his strangely adult comment that it was bad luck.

Loved Objects   *29 December 1985*

Christmas is difficult because it is a time of loved objects. It is not easy for the blind person to take part in this unwrapping, this unveiling of loved objects. It also takes the blind person longer to learn to love that object.

What are the loved objects in my life? I used to love books. I used to love handling my small collection of eighteenth-century books, noting the antique lettering, glancing at the woodcuts or the engravings, and musing over the old handwriting which is often found inside the covers. When I have a new book these days, I certainly like to feel it. I get a certain amount of information from this and I will probably be able to identify that particular book the next time I touch it on my shelves. I always enjoy the smell of a new book, as I thumb the pages. I do not think, however, that I can honestly say that the book becomes a loved object.

Has the love of books transferred to the love of tapes? Hardly! Nobody loves cassettes the way people love books. Cassettes lack individuality and immediacy. The cassette has little or no personality until you put it on the deck. Then it speaks to you, but a new book speaks to you the moment you pick it up. The love for the book requires no mediation from a machine.

I used to love gramophone record covers. I used to admire the artwork, the way in which the atmosphere of the music was often so cleverly suggested through the illustration on the sleeve. Today, the sleeve is merely a casing, merely a protection for the disc and something upon which to put the braille label. Apart from this, the record covers are indistinguishable one from the other.

And what about people? Are not even people becoming indistinguishable? Did I not wonder if it was Lizzie on my knee? Did I not fail to recognize even Marilyn when she called out in the street the other day? What is the status now of a person as a loved object in my life? Perhaps this is one of the reasons for the boredom of the blind, or at least of this blind person. Should I be taking more active steps to fill my life with objects that I can love, objects the loving of which lies in the feeling of them?

In many ways, the blind person lives in a world which is strangely devoid of objects. A sighted person walking through a city centre comes away with impressions of many hundreds of objects, arranged in shop windows, so as to arouse desire. The blind person walks this route with little or no conception of any of these attractive objects and not many things draw you out of yourself, into life.

Living with a Disabled Body: *1 January 1986*
The Hope for a Miracle

I have been reading the philosopher Maurice Merleau-Ponty's *Phenomenology of Perception* in order to understand what it is to be disabled. He has an interesting discussion about the experience of the 'phantom limb'. People who have had a limb or part of a limb amputated sometimes report that they can still feel the missing limb. They complain of pain or irritation in it. They have sensations of moving it. Merleau-Ponty considers this in relationship to the way in which our whole self-image, our entire experience of being a self, is modified by having the kinds of bodies we do have, whereby we relate to this particular world, a world within which and for which these particular bodies of ours have evolved.

It is through the normal body that we establish involvement with the world. We think of ourselves as playing the piano, going for a walk, meeting a friend, doing the ironing, working out a problem on the computer, and all of these projects involve us as bodily creatures in particular relationships with our environment. It is these worldly-bodily projects which undergo a transformation in the case of the disabled person. He or she, however, refuses to relinquish the world and to abandon the projects. There must be some assurance, some hope, that however severely disabled I may be, I still belong to this world, this familiar world of hopes and plans with which my life has been intertwined these many years.

My awareness of having a body in relationship to this world becomes buried deep within my life. The person involved in writing an essay is absorbed in the act of thinking and writing. The thought that there must be a hand in order to write, fingers in order to hold the pen, eyes in order to see the paper, shoulders in order to attach the arm to the body and so on, will not normally be uppermost in consciousness. How could it be? To get on with one's life in the world, one must take for granted the conditions for that life. For the disabled person, absorption in the world is not so easy, because certain tasks have become more difficult, or even impossible.

The problem for the disabled person is that the ordinary, habitual body, which relates us to the world, is no longer the same as the actual body. This knowledge is unacceptable, because one would be exiled from one's world. The phantom arm, Merleau-Ponty argues, is thus not a mere recollection, but a genuine phantom. The patient feels it now. Refusing to consign an arm to the past, he or she does not merely reminisce about the arm, but experiences life with the arm.

This action, however, confines the disabled person to the past. One represses the fact that the world can no longer be manipulated in the familiar way. The past, the time when one had a whole body, remains the 'true' present. The disabled person cannot expect to adjust to the memory of the accident or illness which caused the disablement, as other sad losses in life. The moment of disablement is not one painful memory amongst others, but represents a change in the world itself, which is negotiated and understood through the whole body. The body which remains buried within consciousness, and is the assumption behind every project, is the whole body. What the disabled person remembers is not so much the accident as the world before the accident, and that past becomes blurred into this present. Authentic first-person experience gives way to a kind of abstract relationship with a body and a world which can no longer be actual for the disabled person. One lives on a former experience, on the memory of having had the memory. So deeply imprinted into us are the stereotypes of our bodily action in the world, that we never really escape from them. The phantom limb is thus a kind of magical act, in which the past is rekindled and the lost body is restored.

In this analysis by Merleau-Ponty we find the key to the vulnerability of the disabled person to promises of magical and miraculous healing. Belief in miracle is for many a disabled person, and for those who love him or her, a way of rationalizing denial of the present. It is a rationalization which is all the more compelling because it may appear to be sanctioned by religion, and is reinforced by the self-accusation and the guilt, the passivity and the sense of having been chastened which many religious people feel, when they are disabled. The poignant tension between past and present time (the real heart of the emotions of disability) is suppressed beneath a highly charged religious expectation which hopes for the reversal of the sequence. By a miracle, the able-bodied past will become an able-bodied future, and the present pain will become a thing of the past.

The real miracle takes place when a disabled person is enabled to shatter the normal world through understanding his or her own shattered body. The real miracle takes place when the new reality is grasped, and the illusion of a physical miracle is overcome. This real miracle of acceptance and transformation creates a new coherent world for a body at home in that world. The problem then is how the new world, the state of being blind or paralysed, relates to the other world, that in which sighted or mobile people live. Without this negotiation between the worlds of the disabled and the able-bodied the disabled person, hoping for a physical miracle, continues to live in a broken world, an experience of contradiction and frustration.

Getting to Know the House   *2 January 1986*

I walked right through the house from the back door to the front door only touching the walls once or twice. I just seemed to know when to step sideways, when to move forward. The house is an extension of my body. It is like a skin, something within which I can move and which is appropriate for the proportions of my body.

We had been living there for three years. It was odd that it should have taken so long to develop that kind of knowledge of the house. Sighted people make a house their own within a few seconds but for me to get that sense of comfort it had taken all this time. The blind person observes his body, while the sighted person observes the house. The sighted make the house an extension of the body through sight but are not aware of doing so. They are not aware of the sensations at the back of the retina which guide them. They do not have to stare around the house; they just go here and there. They do not think about going from room to room but about what will be done when they get there. They are aware not so much of movement as of purpose in moving.

The blind person, on the other hand, is aware of the muscular tension which tells him or her how many steps he or she has taken and where the walls now are. After so many steps, I need to reach out and touch. This will enable me to make a course-correction and take the next few steps. There is likely to be a door open and evasive and protective motions must be made.

Sighted people live in the room, not in their eyes; blind people live in their fingers, not the room. Just as the top of your head feels sensitive when you suspect that the ceiling will fall in, just as there is a tingling in your back when you think someone is following you, so the whole of a blind person's body feels in a strange house.

The reason it took me so long was that I had to work out, by repetition, ratios between the scale of my bodily movements and the scale of the house itself. So many times the reach of the body would bring me to such and such a place. The body itself became a unit of mobility. This was the first house I lived in but never saw.

Blind Babies   *3 January 1986*

Blind babies lag behind sighted babies in several aspects of their development, according to a study by Selma Frailberg (*Insights from the Blind:*

177

Comparative Studies of Blind and Sighted Infants). Blind babies do not stretch out to grasp objects. They not only have blind eyes; they have blind fingers. It is true that the eyes of the blind baby are its fingers. It is the whole body which is blind.

Blind babies do not stretch out their hands towards toys which make noises. Why should they? Merely hearing the noise offers no idea that there is something there which can be touched. It is the sight of the thing making the noise which encourages the baby to believe that there is something there which can be touched. Even sighted babies do not reach out to unveil an object making a noise but hidden behind a cloth until the last part of the first year, failing to realize the physical reality of objects which announce themselves only by sound. The blind baby continues to believe in the insubstantiality of merely sounding objects for some time.

For the sighted baby, it is the image of the object which provides the bridge between the memory of what the thing sounds like and the memory of what it felt like when it was touched. When the thing cannot be touched and is silent, its appearance offers confirmation of its continued existence and availability. For blind babies, there is nothing for the experiences of touch and hearing to be embedded in, nothing to hold them together. It takes the blind baby many months to overcome this developmental problem, to associate audibility with tangibility.

This raises some questions about the nature of the world for the recently blinded adult. Whenever such a person hears a sound, he or she attaches a visual image to it. Sounds of traffic convey images of buses and trucks moving along the street. Unable to use sight to build up a pictorial image of his environment, one makes do with using sound in a visual way. This soon becomes unsatisfying, because of the lack of correspondence between the acoustic world and the visual world, and because of the insubstantial and intermittent nature of sound.

What the blind person must do, if he or she is not to become trapped in a state where present experience is inauthentic because of a refusal to forget the past, is to overcome the desire to attach visual objects to sounds. You must begin to accept sounds as sounds, and not as clues to sights. This is an extremely disturbing and demanding cognitive feat. You must allow the visual image, as the ground in which the link between sound and touch is embedded, to be dissolved. Irresistibly experiencing this dissolution, this growing disconnectedness, one experiences the falling apart of the world, the strange and disturbing sense that there is nothing upon which the various bits of the acoustic and tactile collage can be affixed. The blind adult is experiencing an extremely primitive form of regression, back to the very first months of life, before the bond between the senses was established. One is having to pass through the developmental experience of the blind baby by means of a vast and painful detour which involves the unlearning of one's whole life in the world. Such basic cognitive regression is bound to place the adult under considerable strain, especially when accompanied by the helplessness and other aspects of blindness.

The trick is that one must no longer strain to look through one's ears, but simply to listen with them. So great is the loss of the eyes that the other senses get sucked into the vortex. One has to learn, however, that the ears cannot act as substitute eyes. No sense can substitute for another sense. It is just because of the striking contrast between the seen world and the heard world that it is so difficult to put them together. It is a tribute to the remarkable genius of nature that when the world of sight and the world of sound have been made coherent by the intelligence of perception, the resulting coherence is so effective that we become entirely unaware of it, taking it for granted as the way the world is, not as an achievement of human development. This coherence is destroyed by the loss of one of the senses.

Door knockers which are heard and door handles which are touched are both embedded in doors. Sight is like the door itself. When sight is destroyed, that which is heard and that which is touched fall apart in the most distressing and incoherent way. The most vivid expression I know of this is that once when I was listening to the ringing of a bell I walked into a lamppost. The acoustic world comes and goes but offers no resistance to the body. The acoustic world is full of movement and activity but it is all insubstantial. Littered here and there through it, however, like disconnected and unexpected lumps, are lampposts. They have no place in an acoustic world and are unrelated to it, unrevealed by it. They are on another, disconnected plane of reality. As a blind person I became used to moving through an acoustic world, while remaining ignorant of many of its features. I hear the sound over there, but it could be so many things. In the mean time, there is this tree trunk, this brick wall, which makes almost no sound when I strike it with my hand.

This is why the other person occupies a position of unique importance in the world of blindness. Here the blind person encounters an object which is resistant to his or her own body, not perhaps as painfully as a lamppost, but nevertheless with a certain impact of material substance. At the same time, this encountered object gives out sounds, which do not come and go arbitrarily, and sounds which are beyond the blind person's power to produce. I can slap the lamppost with my hand and there is a sound. I can slap your face with my hand and there is a sound. But the sound you make when you scream is quite different. Both are the result of my action, so why is the scream so much more impressive than the sound of the slap? The sound of the slap is involuntary and places you merely in the world of nature. Your scream, and even more, your expostulation, place you in the world of persons. Eliciting the voice of another person in response to my own voice is an extraordinary acoustic experience. There is nothing quite like it. The substantiality of things that sound is, for the blind person, rooted in the experience of the human voice as coming from the human body. This must be the initial experience of the blind baby. As he or she is held in the mother's arms, the first connections between sound and touch are established.

This gives us a deeper insight into the need of blind people for intimate contact. The way in which people without sight live very close to other people is not only due to their vulnerability, ignorance and need for guidance and help. It is because the coherence of sound and touch, upon which the unification of the blind person's world rests, is rooted in experience of other people. You are my world.

Blindness as a Way of Being in the World   *4 January 1986*

Maurice Merleau-Ponty distinguishes between two kinds of consciousness. Representational consciousness consists of the images or the representations of all the things which our senses inform us about, like a mirror stored with the memories of the representations of the things we have seen. Intentional consciousness, however, is to be thought of not so much as a way of thinking but as a way of being. It is a movement towards a reality, a world of which we ourselves form part. Thus, I do not so much conceive of space and time as belong to them. The knowledge which we have of our bodily movements is not the same kind of knowledge as the knowledge of the world which is disclosed to us by our bodies. When I gain a better idea of a house by walking around it, my attention is occupied by the house, of which I am gaining knowledge, and not by my body, the movements of which I know about, but at a different level.

What is called the body-image is, Merleau-Ponty suggests, merely a conglomerate of all the various equivalences between the body and the tasks which are performed in the world. My body image is not merely a matter of knowing what my body looks like, and having in my mind a corresponding image, but is a matter of knowing how my body is in the world, based upon all the things I know I have done and can do.

These suggestions from Merleau-Ponty make me think that I was wrong in believing blindness to be significant mainly because it plunges one into ignorance about the world. The supply of images which consciousness can mirror is suddenly cut short. I now begin to see that blindness is something deeper than this, something more radical. It is a disruption of the fundamental nature of being in the world, in a way that goes deeper than concepts and images. Before blindness is in thought, it is in life. It is a kind of relationship.

When a child is learning how to reach out for something, it does not look at its hand but at the object of its desire. When an adult wants to grasp something, he or she does not calculate the distance by comparing the length of the arm to the distance of the object and working out if it will reach. You simply reach out to see if you can grab it or not. We don't so much measure space as realize it by being rooted within it.

This helps me to understand why I sometimes feel that I have become a ghost. One loses the body when one can no longer move freely to fulfil one's intentions in the world. It is not simply that the world becomes unreal when one is not able to see it any longer; one's own body becomes unreal because it is no longer plunged into a familiar world.

As a blind person becomes familiarized to his or her new body and new world, various changes take place. Merleau-Ponty describes the white cane as becoming no longer an object in itself, but an extension of the body, providing a parallel to sight.

Seeing with the Whole Body   *1 February 1986*

The whole body is the organ of perception. Merleau-Ponty illustrates this thought by describing how we come to conceive of a cube. We walk around the cube, either physically or mentally. The movement of our body, whether real or imagined, is an intrinsic part of the experience of cubeness. We may, of course, turn this experience into a sentence, a definition about six-sidedness and so on, but the moment we try to conceive of the cube itself, we must take up a point of view towards it, imagining that we are inside it, or outside it. This is because our own bodies are always either inside or outside any particular cube. We always see cubes from a particular perspective. A cube without perspective would be a cube as it is for itself, but the cubes we see are never for themselves, but always the cube as seen from our perspective, the cube for us. If one tries to think of the cube from no particular point of view, the structure of the cube is destroyed.

All of our external perceptions relate to some part of the body itself. My body is one further object in the world, as can be seen by the fact that if you ask me where my hand is, I do not say 'It is on the table next to the book, about six inches in from the corner,' nor do I say 'It's on the end of my arm'. The question about the location of my hand is not the same as a question about the location of an ordinary object in the world. At the same time, objects in the world are equally related to my body, and are modified by the conditions which my body imposes upon my perceptions.

This leads us on to a consideration of the seeing body in contrast to the touching body. A seeing place and a seen place are not the same as a touching place and a touched place. Merleau-Ponty points out that for the sighted person all tactile impressions are secondary to visual impressions.

When the sense of touch is modified by the loss of sight, its entire function undergoes a change. In the normal, integrated experience it is difficult, if not impossible, to distinguish one sense from another with any sharpness. This is because what is experienced through one sense is already modified by the other senses. The normal person feels what sight has taught him or her to expect, and sees what habit (the whole configuration of remembered being-in-the-world) has taught him or her to see. Each sense is a smaller world within a larger one. The experience of unity of space is not a conceptual unity, formed when we put together the dimensions of height, breadth and depth, using our reason. It is a lived unity, created by the integration of the senses in their relationship with the world.

The space which is created by the sense of touch alone is quite different. Merleau-Ponty quotes the experience of adults who have recovered sight after a period of blindness, and have remarked that the sense of space which sight confers is so vast, so luminous and so comprehensive that it makes the sense of space conveyed by touch so little, so vulnerable, as hardly to be called a space at all. This, however, has to be learned by the newly sighted adult. He or she will at first have to run the eyes around the disc of a circle before realizing that it is a circle. In the same way, the fingers would have been run around the edge of a circle in order to identify it as a circle, when the person was blind. So, in the first stages of the recovery of sight, the eye is used as if it were a finger. Each sense explores space in its own way and creates a space of its own kind.

Merleau-Ponty recognizes that the sense of sight is built upon touch, and is a development of touch, considered from the developmental point of view. Nevertheless, there remains a fundamental experience of touch which is not comparable to sight, which has its own distinct mode of being. The essence of the difference between sight and touch is that visual space is presented at the same time, while tactile space is presented bit by bit.

If I am working out the meaning of an embossed pattern with my fingers, it may take many minutes, and often repeated explorations on successive days, to discover what the sighted person will grasp in a split second. It is so difficult to remember the precise detail in the little section which one has just explored with one's finger tips, and to relate it to the bit one is presently exploring. Through gradually increasing familiarity one builds up a picture of the whole, until a theory is formed about what it is. This theory is then confirmed by repeated detailed explorations of first this section, then that section. Even when the object is now thoroughly familiar, and returned to after an interval of weeks, although there is a pleasurable renewal of the acquaintance, there is never the instantaneous appreciation of the whole object which sight alone conveys.

Navigating through the Storm   3 March 1986

This morning I woke up feeling most refreshed, because I had had a beautiful night of dreaming. There was a long series of most exciting adventure stories, all in full technicolour, and I woke feeling strangely purged. My mind had been renewed, had been on holiday, had been in open spaces, knowing the freedom and excitement of living in a visual world.

The most memorable dream took the form of a serial. It was one of those unusual experiences where one wakes up several times, while the dream seems to continue in a series of episodes, in a number of snatches of sleep. It was a sea dream, and the central part, the only section I can remember vividly, showed our party navigating a ship through a wild ocean. We were on the bridge, which was glassed over. Heavy seas were breaking upon this glass roof. The waters were crashing down upon a sort of skylight. We were afraid that the ship would be swamped should this skylight window break. It was shivering and shaking with the great masses of water pounding down upon it. Several of us were stretching up our arms to hold the frame steady in case it should collapse inwards with the force of the water. It did not break and we came successfully through the storm and into port. I awoke with an exhilarating sense of recreation, happy at having had all these wonderful experiences.

Sighted people live in the world. The blind person lives in consciousness. From this consciousness there is no escape, or escape is permitted only occasionally as in dreams. Such escape is blissful.

'Between You and Me, a Smile'   *21 March 1986*

Yesterday morning I was kneeling on the floor, helping Lizzie to get dressed. When she was finished, I stood her up in front of me and said, 'Now! Let's have a look at you.' I held her face lightly between my hands while she stood there, and gave her a big smile.

We remained like that for a moment and then she said, 'Daddy, how can you smile between you and me when I smile and when you smile because you're blind?'

I laughed, and said, 'What do you mean, darling. How can I what?'

With great hesitation, and faltering over every word, she said, 'How can you smile – no – how can I smile between you and me – no – between you and me a smile, when you're blind?'

'You mean, how do I know when to smile at you?'

'Yes,' she said, 'when you're blind.'

'It's true, darling', I said, 'that blind people often don't know when to smile at people, and I often don't know when to smile at you, do I?'

She agreed.

'But today I knew you were smiling, darling, because you were standing there, and I was smiling at you, and I thought you were probably smiling at me. Were you?'

Happily, she replied, 'Yes!'

So this little child, having just had her fourth birthday, is able to articulate the breakdown which blindness causes in the language of smiles. I noticed the fine distinction she made by implication between smiling at someone and the smiling which takes place between people. I cannot describe my emotions as I reflected upon the fact that she had had so many experiences of smiling at me, but that the in-between smile was, for her and me, not only a great rarity, but a puzzle. I had endured a terrible loss and been granted a wonderful gain simultaneously.

'It's Like Going Down and Down'   *20 April 1986*

Thomas and Lizzie were sitting on my knee. I was telling them a story. Thomas began to poke my right eye with his finger. He asked, 'If I do that and that, will your sight come back?'

'No,' I said, 'nothing will make my sight come back.'

'Not ever?' he said. 'When you die, will it come back? Will God make it come back then?'

'Well,' I speculated, 'I suppose that, in a way, when I am entirely in God I will know everything, won't I?'

Lizzie then joined in with an exclamation. 'It's not very nice, is it?' She repeated this again quite emphatically. 'It's not very nice, is it?'

'What?', I asked.

'Being blind,' she cried, 'always!'

I said that it was not very nice, but that there were worse things.

'But it's not very nice!' she insisted passionately.

Again I repeated the thought that there were worse things, but she seemed not to hear me.

She burst out, 'It's like going down and down and down and down and down and down and down to the bottom of a very very very very very very very deep well where you can never get out, like in the castle.' She was referring to a trip we had made recently to the ruins of Ludlow Castle where she had been impressed by the dark depths of the well. We had dropped stones down it and listened. Lizzie shrank away from the edge. Now, with a shudder, she said, 'I didn't like that castle. I don't like that place. I don't like those dungeons, and that going down and down and down and down that well. I don't ever want to go back to a castle like that again.'

I think that by now she had more or less forgotten what it was that had made her think of the castle but I was most impressed by her insight into the blind condition, and her instinctive awareness of the horror of the receding light, of the experience of going deeper and deeper down, of the revulsion and rejection one feels in the presence of an irretrievable loss and at the sense of being trapped in there for ever.

In the Beginning Was the Word   *21 April 1986*

We are surrounded by sound from well before our birth until the moment we die. Periods of sight alternate with periods of lack of sight as sleep and wakefulness alternate, but periods of sound do not alternate with periods of silence, for even in sleep we are still upheld within an environment which is charged with sound. You wake up when the ticking of the clock suddenly stops, when your child's regular breathing can no longer be heard. In our normal social lives we are never without the continual presence of sound, which can thus be regarded as the fundamental holding environment. This has the effect of always placing the brain into a relationship with the surrounding world. The brain is one and the world is one because the brain is aware of being in a world. Sound is the fundamental form of that world.

What would it be like to be born entirely without hearing? Would not the world be experienced as less sustaining, more fragmental, more solitary?

The worlds of blind and sighted people are very different. Nevertheless, there are circumstances in which they are joined. When I hold the one I love in the darkness, half asleep, it does not matter that she is sighted and I am blind. She can, to some extent, enter my world by closing her eyes, and we can to some extent, create a mutual world by turning out the light.

It is much more difficult for the worlds of deaf and hearing people to become reciprocal. One could wear ear-muffs. Nature, however, does not close down our ears, so there is no natural point of correspondence between hearing and deaf people such as is offered to sighted and unsighted people by the closing of the eyes, or equally by the coming of night.

It is more difficult for hearing/sighted people to appreciate the mental processes of deafness than of blindness. The sighted person lives in the world as illuminated by the intentions of consciousness. The blind person lives more intensely in consciousness itself, that is, in the flow of thought in which consciousness reaches awareness. Such thoughts are experienced as internal speech, and internal speech can become external speech. So communion is born.

The deaf person, however, lives in a world illuminated by a different kind of consciousness, because of the different development of the mirroring between consciousness and the world of which language is the medium. It is because of this that one can understand how blindness may be experienced as an enrichment of consciousness, while it is harder to realize how deafness could bring this about. There have been blind seers and deaf speakers but while the latter are credited with amazing skill, the former are sometimes thought to have deeper insight. Is this merely a cultural stereotype?

Every impoverishment has its appropriate spirituality and there are a number of deaf people for whom deafness has become the path to spiritual enrichment. I continue to believe, however, that the processes which result in this enrichment are more mysterious. In the beginning was the word.

A Crack in Consciousness   *25 April 1986*

The West Edmonton Mall in Alberta is more than a big, covered shopping centre. It is one of the finest products of the consciousness-creating industries, an environment almost totally controlled in the interests of consumerism. Its many hundreds of shops, some of which are in themselves large department stores, are set in spacious, pedestrian boulevards. You can take a submarine trip to see sharks in the sea which is visible over the balcony of the mezzanine floors. You can observe the full-scale reproduction of a Spanish galleon.

As an all-encompassing acoustic environment, I found it fascinating. Real waves came foaming in on the beaches of the inland swimming sea (not the same as the one with the sharks), while the roar of the crowd watching the ice-hockey match came floating along from some distant part. Around this corner one came upon a brass band, here was a jazz band and over there, several blocks along, a school children's orchestra of recorders and drums. Now there were the screams and the metallic shrieks of the fairground equipment, and the shudder as the carriages on the two roller-coasters went shooting past within a few feet of my face. Everywhere was the endless clatter and tramp of feet; children's feet running and skipping, the brisk patter of women's heels, the steadier tramp of boots and the lighter hesitancy of the feet of old people. Above everything there was the incessant noise of the fountains, tuned to rise higher and so increase in volume as the crowds increased, and to drop down and thus be more quiet when the arcades were more deserted. There were almost no seats. You were expected to keep moving, and the heightened noise of the fountains is said to encourage the crowds not to loiter.

It was a wonderful place. The children would have loved it. I wished they were there. They could have played all day. My feet hurt. I wished there were somewhere to sit down. I wished I could find a quiet place. What was this all about? What were they trying to do to us?

We went to the men's washroom. As we passed through the door, the temperature dropped slightly and the door swooshed shut behind us, leaving us in a different place. It was completely silent. Well, almost completely silent. There were a few noises appropriate to the place, but the surprising thing was that one could hear them so distinctly. It had a quality of stillness, and I realized that whoever made the West Edmonton Mall made a mistake in the design of the men's washroom. They should have broadcast the noise of the open mall into this little place. As it was, they had created a contrast. There was a crack in the all-pervading

187

consciousness. It was like a chapel. We leaned against the walls, enjoying the quiet murmur of each other's voices. We consulted our watches. We said, 'Let's go home.'

When I came to Calgary as a partially sighted person, some years ago, I could just make out the white-clad heights of the Rocky Mountains on the horizon with the aid of the telescope on the observation floor of the tallest building. This time, since I could not renew that memory, I wanted to replace it with something else. Some friends arranged for me to visit a nearby Hutterite agricultural colony.

This was a fascinating experience. I adopted an energetic hands-on approach to the buildings themselves, especially the beautifully laid out kitchen, refectory and chapel, and I had plenty of opportunity for quite deep conversations with some of these remarkable people, who have preserved their religious traditions intact since the middle of the sixteenth century. They still speak with the German accent of their Protestant homeland, and read the sermons of their founders in church every Sunday. They offer another sort of crack in the consciousness of modernity.

It did not seem to worry me during this Canadian trip that I could not go sightseeing in the literal sense, and I was not aware of blindness being a problem in the work I was doing. Blindness is a crack in consciousness.

Is Blindness a Gift?   *26 April 1986*

In recent weeks the thought has been in my mind that blindness could be a gift. I cannot quite remember where I got this idea. It may have been through hearing a programme about meditation in which the expression used was 'the gift of silence'.

I resist this thought, for if blindness is a gift, I would have to accept it. I have said to myself that I would learn to live with blindness but I would never accept it.

Yet I find the thought keeps coming back to me, and arouses my curiosity. Could there be a strange way in which blindness is a dark, paradoxical gift? Does it offer a way of life, a purification, an economy? Is it really like a kind of painful purging through a death? Am I to expect that I shall enter into a new, more concentrated phase of life because of this gift?

The philosopher Brentano did a lot of his creative work after he lost his sight, and attributed this to his blindness. Should I begin to think of myself not as a person disabled by a defect but empowered by a capacity?

If blindness is a gift, it is not one that I would wish on anybody. It is not a gift I want to receive. It is something which I would rather like to give back, but one which I find I cannot help accepting. A gift you cannot help receiving is rather a strange kind of gift. I suppose that I need feel under no bond of gratitude if I am given something which I cannot help but accept.

Accepting the Gift   28 April 1986

On Sunday 27 April I went with Michael to Mass in Notre Dame Cathedral in Montreal. The service was entirely in French, but it caught my attention. Although I hardly understood a word, I was rapt throughout the whole service.

The organ is one of the most famous in North America, and it certainly was a powerful and beautiful sound. I found myself thinking again about blindness as a gift. As the service proceeded and as the whole place and my mind were filled with that wonderful music, I found myself saying, 'I accept the gift. I accept the gift.' I was filled with a profound sense of worship. I felt that I was in the very presence of God, that the giver of the gift had drawn near to me as one who hardly dares to look upon the result of his work. I felt that he had paused, for a moment, and that soon he must be about his own strange work in worlds beyond my imagining. God had, as it were, thrown a cloak of darkness around me from a distance, but had now drawn near to seek a kind of reassurance from me that everything was all right, that he had not misjudged the situation, that he did not have to stay. 'It's all right,' I was saying to him. 'There's no need to wait. Go on, you can go now, everything's fine.'

We walked to the front and received the bread. This is also a strange gift, I thought. Is not the strangeness of this little wafer of the same kind as the strangeness of that other gift? This also is broken, and it breaks those who eat it. As long as I have God's bread within me and God's cloak around me, I will live in God, and God in me.

Carousel   3 May 1986

The Saturday night following our visit to Notre Dame Cathedral, Michael and I saw a performance of the musical *Carousel* by Rogers and Hammerstein, given by the older pupils in an independent Catholic high school in Edmonton, Alberta. During the interval, Michael read to me a poster which was displayed on one of the noticeboards. It went something like this: 'Perhaps the thing which we have to learn from Christianity is this: that in return for this gift we have nothing to offer.'

I found this a strange thought. The motto was directed to people who thought that they would have to repay something in return for having received the gift. It was intended to tell them that this would not be necessary. Just because it is a gift, there can be no question of a repayment.

In my case, the effect was the opposite. It had never occurred to me that in accepting the gift I should give something back. I had been taking it for granted that no gift in return was expected. The poster made me wonder whether this assumption was justified. Of course, a gift does not require a payment, but reception of a gift places one in a relationship with the giver in which an exchange of gifts is courteous and appropriate.

But what gift could be an appropriate exchange for the gift of blindness? What could I give, what would I want to give which could match the numinous darkness and the brilliantly destructive qualities of blindness?

This morning I attended Mass with my friend Ric Laplante at his local parish church. The reading from the gospel was taken from the farewell discourses of Jesus to his disciples, as recorded in the Fourth Gospel. It included the sentence, 'My gift is my peace which I leave with you.'

These words came home to me with particular force. In thinking that the gift is blindness, perhaps I am not being quite accurate. Blindness is the wrapping, or the medium. The gift lies deeper, on the other side of blindness.

All and Nothing   ·10 May 1986

If blindness is a gift, then death is a gift. What shall we give in return for our death? Whatever we are able to give, it must be in anticipation, for when we receive that final gift, we will have nothing left to give.

But if blindness is a gift and death is a gift what have we to fear? If life is death, then death is life. If darkness is light then light is darkness. The conscious and the unconscious lives are one. We have nothing, yet we have everything. The world, life or death, or the present or the future, all are ours, and we are God's.

12

Touching the Rock

Summer 1986

'You'll Have to Pray to God Then!'   *14 May 1986*

During breakfast yesterday morning Lizzie asked abruptly, 'You've got eyes so why can't you see?'

'My eyes don't work.'

'You'll have to pray to God then!'

'Well,' I replied rather hesitantly, 'perhaps God has ideas of his own about all this. He's not just there to look after us, you know. God's got his own problems.'

'Yes,' Thomas echoed. 'God's got his own problems.'

I added, 'We're here to help him, he's not there just to help us.'

In bed this morning she cuddled up very close to me and whispered softly, 'Can you see just a little bit?'

'No,' I said, 'not even a tiny bit.'

'Oh,' she said.

Teaching Lizzie to Read   *17 June 1986*

I realize now that you do not have to have sight to teach a child to read, although this problem caused me much distress in the early years of blindness, when Thomas was little.

About a week ago I began to take Lizzie into my study before breakfast. She has several sets of flash cards which she is learning to recognize, and a number of books, which she will be able to read when she can recognize all of the cards. She sits on my knee, while I pass each card to her, one by one. If she can tell me what it is, I lay it down on the table. If she is not sure, I ask her to spell it to me. Often she can do this, and she can at least tell me how many letters the word has. Usually, she can tell me enough to enable me to recognize the word. If there is any remaining doubt, or if we get stuck, I can get out the set of letters of the alphabet carved in wood and go through them until she recognizes the initial letter of the word. Often it is easier for her to run out and ask an older member of the family what the word is. We arrange the words in various patterns, forming silly sentences. She loves this and we laugh a lot. I ask her to take my finger and point to each word laid out on the table, and then read them to me again as I replace them in the box. Each day, I narrow down in a special pile the words with which she has difficulty. Each day the number of times we have to ask somebody else gets less. Finally, out comes a book, and with great excitement, off we go. One of the good things about this procedure is that the child has to do all the thinking, all the recognition. She has to help me, and my role as a knowledgeable adult is reduced to a minimum. Instead, I become the friendly, encouraging companion, the one with whom to play.

Two Daughters   *22 June 1986*

I had two separate dreams. Each involved a recovery of sight, and each a daughter.

I dreamed that I was actually in my office. Imogen was helping me. She was typing at a far table. Gradually, I became aware of the fact that I was seeing light. The light increased, turned into a sort of glowing mist, into blurred and then into sharper outlines. Colours gradually emerged. I could see. I could see Imogen's face, on the other side of the large office, as she worked at the typewriter. I was stunned and sat there for some time, without saying anything or moving. Then I got up, and told her what had happened. She was not surprised, but continued to work, saying how nice it was. I went into an adjacent room, opened up some filing cabinets, and got out some magazines, looking at the pictures to make sure that I really could see. It was amazing. I really could. So the dream ended.

The second dream followed immediately. I was playing with Lizzie on my knee. Suddenly, with amazement, I realized that I could glimpse the outlines of her head, and then her face, and then I had perfect vision of her. The first thing I noticed was her eyes. They were brown and enormous. She was not looking at me, but her eyes were darting around, here and there. I noted with wonder the many tiny movements made constantly by the eyes. It seemed incredible to me. Then I noticed that this was only happening in one of her eyes. The other eye was immobile. At that moment, I caught her attention. I saw her good eye widen with surprise as she realized that I was looking at her. We clung to each other. Then I said to her, 'What happened to your other eye, Lizzie?'

'I can't see in that eye, Daddy,' she replied.

'I didn't know. How long? When did that happen? I've never heard that. Why didn't you tell me?'

She said, 'Mummy knew. Mummy knows. Mummy will tell you.'

I went over to Marilyn. 'What happened to Lizzie's other eye?' I asked.

'Oh,' she said, 'that happened a long time ago.'

In the dream, I was overcome by a feeling of intense anxiety about Lizzie's other eye. So I awoke.

I woke up very slowly, groping with the realization that it had been a dream, and then remembering, further back, that I had had an earlier dream, the one about Imogen.

Hello, Goodbye   *4 July 1986*

At a recent conference I was waiting in the foyer to receive the distinguished visiting speaker and his wife. There was a crunch of tyres on the gravel drive as the escorting cars arrived, and a whispered warning told me that the official car was following. Two or three of us lined up to form a welcome party, and a moment later our guest was shaking my hand. The host continued, 'and this is Mrs — '. I stretched out my hand again, and this time tapped something rather bristly. A round of laughter covered our embarrassment as I was informed that I had knocked our speaker on the chin. He had been stooping down, I gathered to help his wife. She seemed to be much shorter. Covered with confusion, I tried again. 'No,' a warm and friendly voice said, 'I'm down here!' I made a sort of mid-course correction and there she was, in a wheelchair. The farewells were not much better. I got slightly confused about where everyone was. Believing that I was shaking him by the hand, I thanked our guest for coming, only to find that I was in fact saying goodbye to one of my immediate colleagues, who had taken my hand merely to bring me over to our visitor. We parted as we had met, with mutual amusement and misunderstandings.

Town Hall   *26 July 1986*

Last night I dreamed that I was speaking at a large conference, in a town hall. For a while, I was on the stage. A number of my colleagues were there. There were vivid, visual impressions of the auditorium. The wide gangways had been furnished with tables for the discussion groups. I spent some of the time sitting in the body of the hall, and some on the platform. I had to be very careful going up and down the steps, and in locating my chair. I was aided from one point in the hall to another by various colleagues, but did not seem to be carrying a white cane.

In considering the extent to which I acknowledge myself as a blind person in these recent dreams, it is necessary to distinguish between the visual quality of the dream itself, and how the dream pictures me. It is the dream that sees me, and what the dream sees (with various degrees of ambiguity) is me as being blind.

The fact that I am seen by the dream, and, indeed, that everything in the dream is seen by the dreamer, is no failure to acknowledge that I, who appear as part of the content of the dream, am blind. It is not I who see the auditorium, but the dreamer. I am seen as having difficulty in getting up and down the steps. I don't see the steps, but the dream sees them, and sees that I don't see them. The sleeping dreamer, who is sighted, admits that the waking person, who is dreamed about, is blind. This does not mean that my subconscious does not acknowledge my blindness, for one always dreams of what one knows, what one senses, or images. The point of view of the dream is different from that of the conscious person, because the dream expresses its knowledge in symbolic or image-like impressions and snatches of memories. When I stand on the platform in real life, I know that down there there are rows of chairs with gangways and people. This knowledge is abstract, in the sense that these thoughts are present in the form of sentences. I do not particularly imagine it, unless someone happens to remark that there are, for example, heavy red curtains hanging around the sides, in which case irresistibly an image flits into the conscious mind. In the dream, however, the sequence of sentences, the running tide of thoughts expressed in language, which more or less fills waking time, is suspended in a series of images, events and emotions in which what is known is directly experienced, not mediated through the abstractions of language. You might be watching a video which showed a conference of blind people, but could you tell, by looking at the film alone, whether the camera person was also blind?

I do not see how the dreamer can cease to see unless the dreamer ceases to know. Perhaps it is significant that I cannot remember having dreamed about people's faces for a long time.

In the dream about the town hall conference, I was aware of other people; of the colours of their suits and dresses. I had a general impression of them being there, in their bodies, visually but without faces, although I knew who they were. How did the dreamer know who these people were? The dream was not particularly auditory, so recognition was not by means of voice. The dreamer has ways of recognizing people without knowing what their faces look like. Will the day come when the dreamer will discover ways of knowing that people are scattered around in space, here and there, without representing them bodily, as blobs of coloured presence?

The Terrible Gift   *27 July 1986*

Since April I have been working through the idea that blindness should be thought of as a gift, in some strange way. Since then, I have noticed many examples of this idea in legend, folklore and religion.

The Amrit ceremony is the rite of admission into the Sikh Khalsa, the dedicated Sikh brotherhood. The Amrit bowl is full of sweet water. The initiate will drink some of this, and some will be sprinkled on his hair and beard, and used to anoint his face. The ceremony is watched by five members of the Khalsa, each armed with a long, ceremonial sword. This is in memory of the incident in 1699 when the Khalsa was founded. The first five faithful disciples offered themselves up for execution by the Guru Gobind Singh, only passing into the sweetness of the Amrit through that terrible ordeal.

This combination of sword and sweetness in the one ceremony is a characteristic feature of this idea of the terrible gift. Many religions express this, and in many different ways. I have recently come across the book by C. S. Lewis called *A Severe Mercy*. This is another variation on the same theme.

Iona Abbey   *22 August 1986*

At first, I found the Abbey buildings very confusing. I was so dispirited by the labyrinths (as they seemed to me) of corridors and stairways, pillars and porches that I could hardly summon up the will to leave the bedroom. I found it impossible to learn the layout of the place, because every time I set foot outside the door of our room, kind-hearted people gave me such a lot of help that I could not take anything in.

After two or three days of this I changed my tactics, venturing out late at night when everyone was asleep, or during a quiet time of the day when everyone had gone out. Then I would explore.

I learned the routes to the dining hall and the library. Each time I went out, I filled in a few places on the map I was forming in my mind. One night I discovered a very large wooden door. Opening it, I immediately realized I was in some vast space. It was too still to be outside, but the coolness and the movement of the air suggested an enormous area. I must not get lost. I was at the head of a stone stairway. Every time I went down a few steps I would retrace the way back to the door, making sure I could get out again. The stairway seemed to be interminable, although in fact I suppose it was not more than twenty or thirty steps. At the bottom, there was a huge area of stone floor. It was enough for one night. I had discovered the Abbey itself.

Every night I returned, to explore a little bit more. From pillar to pillar I would work my way, counting the steps, remembering the angles, always returning to the foot of the stairway.

After several nights, I discovered the main altar. I had been told about this, and I easily recognized it from the description. It was a single block of marble. Finding one corner, I ran my fingers along the edge, only to find that I could not reach the other end. I worked my way along the front and was amazed at its size. The front was carved with hard, cold letters. They stood out boldly, but I could not be bothered reading them. The top was as smooth as silk, but how far back did it go? I stretched my arms out over it but could not reach the back. This was incredible. It must have a back somewhere. Pushing myself up on to it, my feet hanging out over the front, I could reach the back. I did this again and again, measuring it with my body, till at last I began to have some idea of its proportions. It was bigger than me and much older. There were several places on the polished surface which were marked with long, rather irregular indentations, not cracks, but imperfections of some kind. Could it have been dropped? These marks felt like the result of impact. The contrast between the rough depressions and the huge polished areas was extraordinary. Here was the work of people, grinding this thing, smoothing it to an almost greasy, slightly dusty finish which went slippery when I licked it. Here were these abrasions, something more primitive, the naked heart of the rock.

13

A Fall into Consciousness

Spring/Summer 1991

A Fall into Consciousness   *12 March 1991*

I dreamt I was in a room. A man threw himself through the window and fell to his death on the coast. There was a terrifying glimpse of the enormous height of his fall. I could see the beach and the waves far, far below as he fell towards it 'Oh, dear,' I was thinking, 'the height is too great. He won't survive. Falling into the ocean from this height would kill him; but anyway I doubt whether he'll even hit the water; he'll fall into the waves, on the border of the sand and the ocean.'

Instead of calling the Coast Guard I began to make various arrangements. I was in a meeting, making these arrangements. It occurred to me that I might be criticized for not having called the Coast Guard earlier. After all, there was just a chance he might be alive. Reports started to come in. A helicopter had found the body, crushed, on the rocks, along the seashore.

I woke up. It had been a dream.

Someone had fallen from a great height on to a border between the earth and the ocean, the world of light and air and the world of depth and darkness. Someone else knew this, someone who was carrying on with business. Someone should have felt guilty that this had happened but did not.

A living consciousness witnesses the extinction of a fallen, border-line consciousness, of that consciousness which could not possibly survive, just because it fell upon the border. Its demise, although both shocking and frightening because of the sheer descent, made no difference to the active, watching consciousness. It was, after all, someone else.

I awoke from this dream with a feeling of profound refreshment, as if I had stepped out of a deep, warm bath. My limbs were warm with it. I emerged from it like a swimmer breaking the surface, the drops and rivulets of sleep splashed from my warm body as I bobbed to the surface.

I knew that the unconscious would always be there, waiting to receive me, like a warm bath. I can step into it any time I want. I can rise from it, reborn. Unconsciousness baptises me. I go in and out of it; I pass through its warm waters; I wrap it round and I unwrap it. It is no longer an abyss, an oceanic depth into which I sink, endlessly and remorselessly, a border upon which I must be crushed and lost. It is my refreshment space which I fill; it is the proportions of my body, no larger than my body; it is my coffin, made for my body but I am not afraid of it.

Losing sight has meant a fall into consciousness.

The Rain Porch   *13 March 1991*

I woke up at three o'clock in the morning. Rain was pattering on the bedroom window. I went downstairs, unlocked the interior doors and went into the rain porch. We had recently had this small porch added on to the back of the house. The instructions to the builders were that it had to be noisy; no double glazing, reverberating plastic panels in the roof, tiles on the floor and no soft furnishings. The first heavy fall of rain revealed that it was really not noisy enough, but luckily a couple of the panels in the roof cracked, which gave us an excuse to replace them with sheets of corrugated metal. This was most satisfactory.

As I opened the door to the rain porch the sound hit me, a steady drumming. I found the day bed, which by some remarkable chance was in its place and not left outside in the garden, located a blanket and pulled it over me. As I lay there, I thought of my childhood, of holidays in tents. We were trained not to touch the inside because a trickle of water would run down the canvas. I thought of the various verandas where I had slept as a child, with their iron roofs, fly-wire, and blinds which could be drawn for protection against rain and wind. I thought of my mother and my father. The rain whispered like my mother's voice, singing simple hymns and melodies that she remembered from her own childhood. I felt surrounded by her and by my father's care; surrounded by everything I had been and was.

I thought of the children, asleep upstairs. How good it was to have all five of them there! I thought of Marilyn, asleep. I thought of the different rooms of the house around me, like cells in a honeycomb, built up like boxes, one upon the other, warm and complex, like a hive, each containing its loved objects, its loved persons. I thought of the rain coming down upon the whole house like a blessing. I felt deeply blessed, surrounded by love.

When I woke up, the rain had stopped. The rain porch itself had therefore disappeared; I was just there on the day bed. I went back into the warmth of the main house; it was completely silent, but it breathed in its silence like a living creature. I went upstairs; Marilyn was sleeping peacefully. It was six o'clock, and the first birds were singing.

Drowning in Committee   *14 March 1991*

Each year the University carries out a review of the performance of academic staff, and on the basis of this a small number are selected for promotion to senior posts. The process of selection begins at the departmental level then goes to the faculties, finishing up with a meeting of the seven Deans of Faculty together with the Vice-Chancellor and the Pro-Vice-Chancellors. The review process is extremely thorough and highly competitive.

Last year's meeting had not been an easy one for me. I had been Dean of the Faculty of Education and Continuing Studies for less than three months and was still discovering how the systems worked. The week before the crucial meeting I had visited the central office accompanied by an expert reader whose respect for confidentiality was absolutely guaranteed, and spent a whole morning working my way through the papers of the various candidates who were to be presented at the meeting. I was, of course, particularly concerned about how I would present my own candidates, of whom there were half a dozen or so. They had already received a rough grading and I felt pretty confident that the top one or two would be accepted without too much discussion. At a certain point down my list there was bound to be controversy, so I devoted a lot of time to carefully memorizing the details of the candidate who was likely to be the subject of the fiercest contention. Those further down my list I felt fairly sure would not be successful and I did not devote so much time to their papers.

As it happened, the meeting had taken a different direction. I was called upon to speak, not on behalf of the colleague whose papers I had prepared so carefully but on behalf of another one. The order in which the Deans would speak was to be alphabetical, with the Faculty of Arts going first. It was agreed that each Dean would present a number of candidates, roughly in proportion to the size of the Faculty. We were to take notes of each candidate's case and at the end of the speeches and discussion we would be asked to vote. Arts had spoken first, presenting his three or four candidates with an easy and convincing eloquence; next came the Dean of Commerce and Social Science, calm and incisive. I was desperately trying to remember the details of my candidate. Had he written five books or six? Was he the one who had been invited to go as a consultant to UNESCO or was that someone else? I was unable to concentrate on the speeches being made by Arts and Commerce, and I had suddenly realized that I was not going to be in a position to cast an informed vote. I had made my speech, trying to sound knowledgeable, hoping I would not be asked too many questions. There were one or two questions, but fortunately I knew the answers. The meeting moved on to the Dean of Engineering, followed by Law and Medicine and Dentistry. By then we had had fifteen or twenty speeches. I could hardly remember their names, let alone the details. Science was still to come, the largest Faculty of all. The Dean of Science had presented six candidates – a glittering galaxy of brilliant young scientists all deserving of promotion. By then, my mind was nothing but a jelly; names and academic disciplines, titles, medallions and honours ran through it like goblins, disappearing as soon as they were spotted.

The time for the vote arrived. They passed out sheets of paper and we were asked to write down all the names, giving our vote beside each name, from ten votes for the strongest candidates to one or zero for the weakest. A piece of paper had fluttered down on the table beside me as the clerk walked around; my mind had been racing with possibilities: surely the clerk would come and offer assistance? But no, why should he? They respected me; they would assume that I had my way of doing things; they would wait for my suggestions. All around me the noise of scribbling, heavy sighs of concentration and the occasional cough filled the air. Where had that clerk gone to? Should I attract the Pro-Vice-Chancellor's attention? It was too late. They were gathering in the papers and commencing the count. I had muffed it.

Somebody around the table had said, 'Wait, I don't believe we have John's votes yet.' The Pro-Vice-Chancellor had turned to me and said, 'What would you like to do, John?' I had explained that perhaps on that occasion it would be best if I did not take part in the vote. I had not come completely prepared for the procedure but I would think more carefully about the techniques which could be adopted at next year's meeting. The Chair, obviously concerned and sympathetic, had replied, 'Anything you say, John, we will do anything you think appropriate.'

There had been a dead silence then. Everyone realized that a mistake had been made. No one knew quite what to do about it. I had felt enraged with myself for having allowed this to happen; I should have foreseen some such procedure.

The results had been announced and somebody had remarked, 'Yours got in all right, anyway, John.'

'Yes' I had replied, 'and without my vote.' What would I have done, I wondered, had my candidate been beaten by one or two votes? My vote would have made the difference. I would have had to call upon the Chair to declare the meeting out of order and to take the entire vote again. This would have been the most awful predicament, and I had broken out in perspiration at the thought of it.

At the end of the meeting I had blundered from the room and stumbled down the stairway, striding rapidly across the spacious foyer, not caring if I walked into a marble pillar or not. I had walked across the campus and home in a sort of angry daze, cutting the air and the ground with my cane as if it had been a knife, wishing that I could swish it through walls and posts and cut up the ground itself in front of me so that I could disappear. I had been furious at myself for being blind; I had felt actually angry at the blindness as if it were a personal enemy, an alien power always sitting on my shoulders like the Old Man of the Sea, weighing me down and strangling me wherever I went. If only I could shake the damn thing off!

When I got home, Marilyn had taken one look at me and said, 'What on earth has happened? You look terrible!'

I had told her the story, trying to keep my voice steady. She went mad. 'They didn't behave like that because they respected you!' she had cried. 'They just hadn't thought of it, any more than you had! Nobody gave it a thought beforehand! Why didn't you go and see the Pro-Vice-Chancellor and sort it all out sooner? Why didn't they have the sense to realize they were putting you in an impossible position? Why didn't you stand up for yourself more the moment you realized it? You have got to get a grip on this situation and confront it, otherwise you won't be able to go to one of those meetings again. You will have to make them change the procedures or you will have to find a way of doing it their way.'

I had known she was right. Every word she had said was true, about me, about my colleagues, about all of us. There had to be a way round the two aspects of the problem: information input (I had to have a way of getting at the data when I needed it) and output (I had to be able to take part in the vote).

A Vote of Confidence   15 *March* 1991

The answer to the input problem was braille. I had taught myself braille in a hospital in Melbourne when I was nineteen and had read the Gospel of Mark and some of the Psalms in the hospital. I had not really looked at braille since then, until I became a registered blind person. I had had a braille manual at home, which Marilyn had brought into the Birmingham and Midland Eye Hospital. I had turned over the pages, gently feeling the layout. The inside cover was obviously merely a pattern; it was too repetitive to be a code. What followed must be the title page. There followed a number of pages with braille on the left linked with lines of dots to smaller pieces of braille on the right. These must be the contents pages, but where was the key? Presumably in the first chapter they would set out the braille alphabet in a column. I seemed to turn innumerable pages before I came to it. Finally, I came to a page where individual braille cells were laid out across the page. This had to be the alphabet, and I soon remembered the A and the B. The rest was easy. Within a few days I was reading the Gospel of John, slowly but with enjoyment.

Braille is an extremely simple and logical code. Learning to read braille is like learning to play the piano; you can do it in half an hour, but to get good at it takes years of practice. Although I came to use braille regularly for labelling cassettes and gramophone records, I did no serious reading in braille. It was too slow, clumsy and heavy on space. With cassettes, I was as fast as the sighted reader. With braille, I would never be as fast. Moreover, on cassette I could slip a 500-page book into my pocket. With braille, I would need a forklift truck. I tried to read a bit of poetry and some Bible passages every day, in the hope of gradually improving. I was always conscious of the fact that if I went deaf, I would be dependent upon braille.

Writing braille was a different matter. Braille is an embossed code, and manually has to be written from the back, and thus in reverse. I had bought several braille frames and a stylus and got to work. Within a few days of coming out of the hospital I began to experiment with the labelling in braille of my gramophone record collection. I can remember one evening trying to write Beethoven's name in braille. It was tricky. Sometimes I got the 'th' sign round the wrong way, but if the 'th' was right then I managed to get the 'v' pointing in the wrong direction. I did it twenty-three times. On the twenty-third time it was correct.

The day after the problem on the academic staff review committee, I had made contact with the disability rehabilitation unit provided by the government. A week later, they were in my office assessing my problems. Another week later, I had been equipped with a braille typewriter and a neat little computer with a braille keyboard and synthetic speech, braille or print output. When it came to having an agenda, a set of names or times or details set out before one during a meeting, braille was the answer. Synthetic speech was not the answer, because you could not listen to two things at once. Moreover, there was always a problem of having exactly the right bit of speech available at the right moment. Only a braille spreadsheet could do that.

Getting my contribution back to the meeting would be more difficult. This had to be a combination of careful preparation and common-sense human relationships.

When this year's meeting came round, I prepared the papers on every candidate, not just the one or two I thought I might have to speak about. I memorized the main outline of everybody's curriculum vitae and publications list and made a braille summary of each candidate. I interviewed each candidate separately for one hour, making sure I had a grasp of every detail of his or her work and publications. Every such interview was tape recorded by permission. I listened to these tape recordings before the crucial meeting, summarized them and memorized the summaries. When I went into the meeting, I was bustling with facts right up to the eyebrows.

I arrived at the meeting early and met one of the senior secretaries. I asked him to write down the name of each candidate as the speech was made about that candidate; just the name would be sufficient. As the speeches were delivered, I held in my hand a micro-recorder. I whispered the name of the candidate and immediately gave my vote, thinking that at the end of the series I could revise my vote if necessary. When the speeches were over I intended to re-wind quickly, play the tape back close to my ear and thus give my votes to the secretary.

In the event, I did not have to play the tape back to myself; I vividly remembered each name and each speech; the secretary sat next to me and fired the names at me in a low whisper. At each whisper I shot the votes back to him. The whole process took less than a minute. I think that we were the first to finish. It was certainly several minutes before the secretary got up and started to retrieve the voting papers. Everybody else in the room was puffing and sighing, coughing and shuffling through their masses of notes. Of course, they had to write all the names out, whereas I had the names already written out. Nobody made any comment and I am not even sure that the people noticed what I was doing. It was routine. It worked. I had voted.

The Seasons   *16 March 1991*

I used to think that, having lost my sight, the seasons would mean little or nothing to me any longer. In the winter the trees became quiet; in the summer, they were noisy again. It was cold in the winter, warm in the summer; that was about it.

I have changed my mind. Perhaps my blind mind has become more seasoned. In the first place, when I open the front door and stick my head out, the experience is different according to the season. If it is a very cold winter, it is like putting my nose inside an icebox. The east wind cuts like a dry knife; I have to hold my breath, so sharp is the air in my lungs. When the spring comes, if I put my nose outside the door early in the morning, at half-past-five or six, I feel like a dog. I feel it not only with my nose but with my whole body: the fragrance in the air, the movements of the wind, the odours of growing things, the moisture in the air, the freshness of the dew-laden atmosphere – it is so beautiful. It is not so much that I smell it; rather, I feel it, I sense it all over. It is a different world from the winter world.

Just as in the absence of a specific organ of sight I have become a whole-body seer, so although my organ of smell is intact I have, somehow, become an all-body smeller. Perhaps a generalization of one sense encourages another sense to become less specific. Perhaps if all of our senses were less specific we would become more alive, all over.

Why Is Thunder Like Scratching?   *17 March 1991*

Thunder is like scratching because both create a border for experience. Without a border I am conscience within an infinite space, consciousness without a body, without a world, a god without the benefits of deity. The sudden imposition of a limit to experience, the creation of an experience which tells me 'on this side of the experience, I am; on the far side of that experience I am not' changes me from being a mere reflection into a location. Instead of merely saying 'I am', now I can say 'I am here, not there; I am within these borders, I have a point from which to view, therefore a viewpoint, therefore a self, a finite self, a human self.'

The fact that the first experience is imposed by one's skin, so close, while the other is imposed by the clouds, so distant, does not change the principle of this experience. The clouds are my skin; my skin is a thunder-storm; each takes hold of the mind spinning in space and says to it: Stop. You are here.

Does Your Memory Improve When You're Blind? · 20 March 1991

I have always been sceptical about the claim that the blind have wonderful memories. Certainly, you remember what you have to remember. If you are setting out on a train journey and you know that you will not have access to the arrival and departure times at some crucial point where you have to change trains, except through consulting your memory, you remember the times. Whether there was anything more than that, I was uncertain.

It does seem to me, however, that an increased speed and confidence in memorizing did play a part in the contrast between the two business meetings I have described. One develops techniques without thinking very much about it. Everything has to have numbers and headings. If someone is reading to me fifteen points of an agenda, it is important that the points each receive their number. The number is associated with the topic, and without the labels provided by the numbers the topics become confused. There is also a quality of attention: you listen more carefully and make a point of remembering details which you know you will need and which you will not have another opportunity to get at. So you listen, you think, you rehearse in your mind. A good deal of memory is motivation.

It is easy for sighted people to exaggerate the memory-expertise of the blind. If during a business meeting I refer to sub-section 2b of Item 8, people are rather surprised. They get the impression, which suits me very well, that I have memorized every point in the same way. In fact, I have probably made a special note of that particular item because it was important to me. If they were to respond by quoting some other point in similar detail, I would have to ask them to read it to me. But not all is the result of exaggeration and misunderstanding. I have experienced, particularly in the last six months, an expansion in my capacity to absorb spoken material, and for me spoken material includes both the printed text which is read to me and the lectures and conversations which I hear. It is all spoken word. Somehow or other I have become more retentive. Naturally, sometimes I go to sleep, sometimes I am just not very interested and not even listening; sometimes I try to remember and forget or make mistakes. Nevertheless, there has been a significant expansion.

This has given my brain a new sense of well-being compared with the situation three or four years ago. My brain feels the tension of being in use, as if the net has been pulled tighter, in contrast to the painful, gnawing emptiness, the tension of anxiety and hunger which used to distress me so much. My brain used to hurt; now it feels more used, more cared for and hence happier and more efficient. Whereas my brain was previously starving for facts, it now eagerly seizes any fact, however small, and devours it with enjoyment. When there is a famine of information, every crust of bread is a delicacy to be relished and remembered. So I have learned to love knowledge just as knowledge, and to realize that to know is to be alive.

Acoustic Envelopes   *14 June 1991*

In interactive, multimedia presentations of environmental planning, the expression 'visual envelope' is used to describe the scene as it would appear from a particular point of view or at a particular time. So by pressing the screen one can get the visual envelope now, six months into the construction period, and five years later. One can get the visual envelope from the point of view of any house situated along the edge of the affected area, such as a proposed new rail link. This helps me to think of acoustic envelopes and their effect upon walking.

In the early years of blindness I used to think that walking was boring because you never seemed to get anywhere. There was no anticipation; your legs just kept going up and down, up and down and a certain amount of work would lead to a result. The actual pleasure of moving through an environment had gone, I thought.

I now believe that this was an understandable exaggeration. Once you have learned to bivouac in the acoustic world, you have the experience of passing through a number of envelopes, to mix the metaphors. One could also think of each envelope as being an aural ecology, a world with an intrinsic structure where each sound is not arbitrary but depends upon the rest of the contents of the envelope. The fundamental conditions of each space provide a concatenation of harmonious sounds which, put together, constitute a little world. I pass through five of these during my walk to the office; first, there is the world of the house, second, the suburban side streets, third, the busy highway, fourth, the campus itself and finally, my own building. I will describe these five environments as they appear between 6.30 and 6.45 in the morning.

The house is still but for the sounds of breathing children. The refrigerator hums. The dishwasher switches itself on and off. In the eaves there is the scrabble of birds feeding their young. Throughout the house there is the occasional crack and squeak from woodwork and metal. The curtains rustle as the breeze moves through half-open windows.

The toilet flushes next door. There is a pad of feet as a child runs from its own bedroom to our bedroom. I pull back the bolt with a snap, unlock the front door, click it behind me, unlock the door of the porch and swing it open. The second aural envelope greets me.

I move from enclosure, warmth, fragrance and intimacy into an enormous sense of space. I move like a fish through eddying currents of fragrant morning air; it carries me like a swimmer down to the main road. The wood pigeons are calling; overhead, the rustling trees make a canopy, the taller trees like an awning set high above. I come to the corner of the first block and there is a sweet, cool current of air moving down the side street towards me. The south-westerly is blowing. It is like stepping into a river. Now I have crossed the side street and am on the far side; the river is cut off as I am sheltered by the houses. The road is still, apart from the occasional purr of a car passing; there are no other pedestrians. Still the wood pigeons are calling.

I come to the Bristol Road. I have come down into the valley. The fragrant, moving, morning air up on the hill has gone. Here there is a thicker, more turbulent motion made up of exhaust fumes. Already at this hour, the road is packed with trucks and buses. There is rumbling, roaring, purring, swishing of dozens of different kinds of vehicles. If only I could learn to identify them! I can distinguish the big ones from the little ones. As I wait for the lights to change, there is a taxi with its engine idling, waiting; at least, it is certainly a diesel engine and a small one.

The bleeps begin to sound, and as if the traffic heard it, it becomes silent, respectful, waiting. Through that silence I pass, and the bleeps are all around me, behind me, in front of me. They protect me like bird sounds crying out to the waiting traffic 'Wait, wait, wait!' Now I am over, through the main gates of the University and into the third environment.

I walk across parkland, sheltered from the sounds of the main highway by an embankment. It is cooler; here, the morning sun has not yet penetrated. There is once again a sense of the early morning, rather like that up on the hill. The sound of my cane strikes echoes from the nearby buildings. Above and all around the birds are singing their hearts out. Why are they so joyful? What do they know that we don't know? We know it too, if we would only listen. I climb higher, up the hillside, across the rough ground under the bridge which leads to the University car park and up the steps and there it is again! The south-westerly, strong and steady like a stream of power and fragrance. I plough into it, breathing it in and out. I am one with it.

I turn the corner into the University Ring Road and I am now pursued by a monster. It roars with a deep sucking motion of brushing and rolling as it approaches me. It is the University street-sweeping machine doing its early morning run around the campus. It pauses as I walk past it. Has it seen me or is it just having a fag? I pass through a cloud of heat and mechanical oily smells. Now I am in front of it. It follows me. If I walk fairly steadily I can keep it just about thirty or forty yards behind me. Will it catch me? I am like a child; this has become a silly game. I pause to tighten the end of my white cane. The thing draws closer and closer. The roaring blots out almost every other sound. Off I go and now speed away from it, trailing my cane along the edge of the curb. It makes a steady stone-like rubbing sound. I must make sure that I do not walk into the next lamppost in my haste. On my right I hear the dim roar of the awakening city traffic; the perimeter roads of the University are also pretty busy, quite a number of cars, perhaps technicians reporting for the laboratories, porters and security guards, the occasional academic hoping to get in a couple of hours before the telephones start ringing. There are no other pedestrians. Everyone is in cars. I alone am nestled in this acoustic world. I alone am truly open to it. I leave the Ring Road, turn towards my building, down the steps towards the door. The monster is coming, will it get me before I open the door? I fumble for the key and throw open the side door and I am in. The street sweeper whines as it realizes it has lost me.

I am into another world. Once again, like the home, it is enclosed, but unlike that warm intimacy, it is large, sharp, clean and impersonal. There is a distant smell of paper and polish. My cane brings the entire foyer to life with echoes. My own footsteps speak to me as I approach the lift. There are the metal doors of the lift, the wooden surrounds, the pleasure of those sharp, straight lines, and now I am in the lift. It is little larger than my own body; for some reason, I want to swish my cane from corner to corner to make sure I am alone. The doors close with a hush of excluded air and I am lifted up. There is a pressure under my feet and a gentle reverberation, a click as I pass from floor to floor and the lift delivers me. The doors open obediently, as it were to thank me and offer me the foyer. The lift did its job; it knew what I wanted. The foyer is waiting for me. I am now in the inner recesses of the higher parts of the building. It is much warmer here. Down the steps, into the still but familiar environment of the corridor. And into my own office. There is a hush, the curtains and the carpet create an intimacy quite different from that of the lift or the foyer. There are layers of books, rows of cassettes, familiar objects. The room is warm with the early morning sunlight pouring in. I open the window. Spread out below me, as far as the ear can hear, are all the murmuring sounds of the life of men and women, a carpet rolling away from this window frame upon which I rest my hands. It needs painting; the paint is chipping off. The glass is like a membrane which divides me from that outside world.

Can Sighted and Blind People Understand Each Other? 15 June 1991

On 2 June we had viewed the BBC *Everyman* documentary film about *Touching the Rock*. Although we viewed it with about forty friends and neighbours, making suitable silly noises and cheering at everything, experiencing the film together did re-open old wounds. It pointed up so vividly the different states within which we live. The opening sequences, showing the train driving into the tunnel, the noise and energy, the mechanical irresistibility, that experience of being carried relentlessly into blindness, filled us both with a fresh sense of the painfulness of those terrible years of transition. The dark tunnel under the mountain holds no fears for me any more; I am nestled within it like a bat that has learned to hang upside-down in this subterranean cavern. But this is not Marilyn's world. How could it be?

We talked of the problem of our life together outside the home. 'Thank goodness,' she said, 'that we have had so many children, because it has made the home environment so wonderfully rich and all-demanding. What would it be like, had we been thrown back upon our own resources, just the two of us?' Who knows?

She spoke of what it was like being at dinner parties together. I said that sometimes I had the feeling she was embarrassed about being with me. I told her how a recent dining out experience had made me realize again how all around a blind person there are innumerable little signals and nuances going on all the time, and every action must be interpreted within the context of those myriad relationships of which a blind person can have but little conception. Our family life is like an intact system on a tiny scale; it works, including friends and regular visitors, through habit and acceptance. Bring a complete stranger into that system, be it a child or an adult, and the system becomes conscious of itself. It has to cope with an extraneous factor. If I am taken out of that little world, if I am outside that interpreted system of codes within which I dwell, I am exposed.

Marilyn said it made her feel as if I were saying that there was a kind of sighted conspiracy. 'But,' she explained, 'it wasn't like that in conversation around the dinner table.' She reminded me, 'Every time anyone speaks, everyone reacts in some way; everyone has an expression, glancing either at the speaker or at each other. There is a continual flow of relationship, of mood, of mutuality.'

I am necessarily cut off from almost all of this. It happens through facial expression, body language. Not everything can be turned into an 'ooh' or an 'oh', a grunt or a laugh. On top of this, she has to cope with the understanding smiles of her friends, with those sympathetic glances, the kind looks of pity. I am immune to it all, but she must catch them and somehow fend them off. She must do all this entirely alone, since I cannot participate in that world of human networks.

I am like a submarine, remorselessly ploughing along, having surfaced or just about surfaced especially for this occasion. Marilyn is like part of the strategic air defence, a fast moving pattern of communications which embraces the entire atmosphere, and into which I am only partially locked. She can communicate with the rest of that network, but not with me, except publicly through words which everyone else will hear. Everyone else can use the whispers of body language; she and I must use the loud-hailers of speech.

She said she was sorry if she didn't seem to understand or enter into my pain, but she felt she was six or seven years behind me in adjusting. I explained that I do not have any pain, perhaps a twinge now and again, but for the rest, there is no pain except for her. Perhaps she is behind me in some ways but she is six or seven years ahead of me in others.

She explained that whenever she is out with me the sense of that entire world, including the children, which is closed to me, fills her with such a sense of loss. I tried to explain that what I cannot see means nothing to me; it is past, it is gone. It is elsewhere, in the consciousness of others. I listen to it, to what these people say they experience. I believe them. I listen with the same kind of interest as when people tell me of their religious experiences or their dreams; these are interesting and important things which are happening to them. I try to interpret, to empathize, to understand it from their point of view. Interested though I am, the things these people see mean no more to me that what they dream; what they describe is not the real world, my world; it remains their world.

Then I thought: if the world of what is seen means nothing to me, and if Marilyn is part of that which can be seen, then part of Marilyn means nothing to me. And she, knowing that, will lose part of herself. Therefore, my change of worlds becomes her loss of identity, but whereas I can forge a new identity, she must be ever painfully between the two, half in half out, always the mediator.

This discussion left us both with a deep feeling of estrangement:

always to be bound, as Paul Tillich puts it, to that from which we can never be separated. I wanted to say that beyond this estrangement there is a new being, created by love, but I could not. The birth of that new being is so slow and painful, intermittent, perhaps never realized except in a few bright moments of revelation. In the mean time one senses, not so much through one's own experience but through the emotions and perceptions of another, how great and terrible is the power of darkness.

If it is true, as the old translation of the Bible says, that the light shines on in the darkness but the darkness comprehendeth it not, it is equally true that the light comprehendeth not the darkness. There is an antipathy, a mutual cancelling out. We sometimes think that the light is all victorious and the darkness yields before it but this is not all the truth. They obliterate each other.

14

Beyond Touch

Summer 1991

Crossing the North Sea   *4 August 1991*

'Line nine: please embark now.'

The public address system repeated the message in Swedish as our car began to move forward with the rest of the line. Gaby, now six years old, sat beside me.

'Tell me exactly when we board the ship, will you, Gaby?'

'Not yet, not yet,' he chanted. Then, suddenly, 'NOW!'

I could immediately tell the difference. A couple of metallic clanks marked our progress; the breeze was cut off and its place was taken by the cavernous echoes of engines shutting down and the smell of oils and fumes. We piled out – all seven of us. Lizzie took my hand.

'You have to go along this little ledge, Dad. Step up over a sort of threshold. Now up a sort of metal staircase. It's narrow and steep. I'll go first.'

She placed my hand on the rail and climbed up in front of me. Soon we had found our cabins and were in the middle of a brisk discussion about who should sleep where. Outside, the broadcast voice of the chief steward could be heard welcoming passengers who had joined the *Prince of Scandinavia* at Newcastle for the voyage to Gothenburg, Sweden.

It was almost exactly ten years since I had last sailed abroad with the family. Marilyn and I had crossed from Plymouth to Roscoff in Brittany. Thomas was twelve months old. I had hated it because I felt responsible. I had been keenly aware of my inability to get from one part of the vessel to another and wondered what I would do if Marilyn, who was not very well, should get worse. How long would I be able to look after Thomas? How would I explain where I had left our things?

This time it was so different. My responsibility was to look after the money, the passports, cheque books and credit cards. That was the lot. Outside, the steward was inviting children to make their way to the lounge area on Deck 7 where the Pirate Club was about to commence.

'Off you all go,' said Marilyn. Thomas, Lizzie, Gaby and Joshua rushed from the cabin like a pirate boarding party. I hitched on to one of them as they whizzed past. For a moment I wasn't sure which one, but it didn't matter. They followed the signs to Deck 7 and soon it was all happening.

'Feel my pirate's hat!'

'What address shall we use on the membership application?'

'Oh, no! They won't take Joshua. You've got to be four. What shall we do with him?'

'Put him on my knee,' I said. 'I'll play cards with him.' I had Joshua's playing cards in my pocket. We dealt the cards out on the table. He snapped them up happily, arranged them in piles, announced that he had won and now it was my turn. There were no rules.

When the children, terribly excited, had finally been confined to their cabin, Marilyn and I walked the decks while Imogen baby-sat. It was a perfect environment for blind people. The deck was almost deserted, and with one hand on the rail, I could walk along with ease and safety. The handrail was broad and smooth, although sprinkled with countless pin-pricks due, I supposed, to the wind and the salt. Every few yards the rail turned a sharp corner and there was a rectangular area which must have been something to do with the launching of the lifeboats. Marilyn told me there was a lifeboat above us, and by stretching up my cane I could touch it.

She went below to make sure the children were all right, and I continued to explore the deck. A couple of men walked past me.

'Do you want a hand? Do you want any help?'

'No thanks. I'm just exploring the deck. Is it OK ahead?'

'Yes, you're fine. It's all clear. You can go right to the end.'

The wind was fresh and fragrant. The deck here was damp and the handrail covered with spray. Now and again the wind carried a mist of fine spray over my face. The whole ship was moving, sliding gently this way and that and purring rhythmically under the power of its engines. I had reached a staircase going up, but with a rope hung across it, preventing access. I leant over the rail. Here, towards the stern of the ship, the sea roared like a cataract, spreading behind us like a waterfall from which we were speeding away.

Sleeping in the cabin was like being in the rain porch at home, except that the cascading patterns of sprinkled sound came not only from above, but from all sides and beneath as well. Moreover, it was tactile. The mattress, the side of the bunk, the bedside table, everything was purring with life and pleasure. The ventilation system imposed a kind of breathing upon the deeper rhythm of the heart. The cabin was just the right size for easy mobility, since you were never out of reach of a characteristic fitting. In the middle of the night Joshua got out of his own bunk and came to mine. I scooped him up and put him in with me. He went to sleep again almost immediately, and as I placed my hand gently on his head, it was vibrating too.

In the morning Marilyn said that she rather wished we had paid the extra to have a cabin with a porthole.

'Would you be able to open it?' I asked.

'No. Some of the cabin doors were open and I glanced in. I don't think the portholes do open, but in any case it would make such a difference.'

'Why? What difference could it make?'

'It's hard to explain,' she said. 'Just being able to see outside. The sight of the sky and the sea makes you feel less cooped up. It's hard for a blind person to understand, I suppose. In a way, you are always cooped up. It helps me to understand the sense of claustrophobia which you used to have, and perhaps sometimes still do. I would feel more like spending time in the cabin if it had a porthole, because I wouldn't feel so closed in. Do you feel closed in?'

'Well, not really, especially not on this ship, where space is structured so beautifully and on such a human scale. What I like about the ship is that it is a finite world, unlike the world on land, which seems to be infinite. There is no traffic on the ship and you can't really get lost because you're always on the ship. But I suppose there is some comparison between a blind person's experience of travelling and a sighted person always travelling in a cabin without a porthole. The world that is doing the travelling is the ship itself, the cabin itself. The ship is not exactly travelling through a world, although the rush of the sea is exciting. It isn't a mobile platform from which to view the world; it is intrinsically interesting. It's a bit like being in a car. The car is vibrating and you know it is moving, but it is not moving through anything, unless you lower a window and stick your hand into the wind. The ship is like that, but it is far more interesting.'

North Koster: The Crossing   *5 August 1991*

Thomas took my hand. 'Come and listen to the noise of the engines turning the sea over.'

We swayed across the upper deck, bracing ourselves against the warm but powerful westerly wind. Thomas put my hand on the metal rail and I followed him gingerly down the ladder, rolling and pausing as the ferry pitched and tossed.

He led me to the stern. This ferry, taking us to the Swedish island of North Koster, was a much smaller vessel than the great *Prince of Scandinavia*. Holding the rail, we found that we were directly above the screws.

'It cuts the sea up to about half a metre or a metre deep,' shouted Thomas in my ear. 'The big ship must have cut it up for at least twice that depth. Do you think Joshua would survive if we threw him in?'

'It depends how far we threw him,' I replied, with surgical precision. 'If we just dropped him over the edge straight into it he would be chopped to bits immediately, but if we threw him as far as we could, he might just clear it.'

We were sheltered from the wind, but clouds of exhaust fumes billowed around us, hot and moist with a sort of sickly metallic tang. The churning of the sea varied with the pitching of the ship, as if the screws took a deeper bite as the vessel lunged down, but roared with an empty fury when momentarily lifted by the surge. Above us was a persistent but irregular flapping sound. Surely the ship did not have sails?

'What's that flapping sound?'

'It's a flag; a big one. I think it's the Swedish flag. It's huge! If you stretch your cane up, you can touch it.'

The wind caught the cane and I swayed for a moment. Thomas held my hand and pushed my arm in the right direction. 'There! You've got it.' I felt the cane shudder as the folds of the flag struck it. I returned the blow, striking the flag a couple of times. I could make out the material, but under the pressure of the wind it resisted the cane.

The next time we used the ferry, the flag was not flying, for some reason. I pointed this out to Marilyn, who exclaimed 'How on earth did you know that?'

'Oh,' I said nonchalantly, 'there was no flapping.'

'I'm amazed that you should have noticed that,' she said admiringly. I gave a cool smile, feeling rather pleased with myself.

North Koster: The Island   *10 August 1991*

North Koster is a small island off the west Swedish coast, just south of
the border with Norway. The island is only a couple of miles wide. It
has a permanent population of about a hundred, mostly fishing families
or retired people. There are no cars, no roads, no amusement arcades,
no fun palaces, no discos or coffee bars or nightclubs. The island is
criss-crossed with little paths and scattered with houses and holiday
chalets, forested with a few low rocky outcrops. The sound of the sea
and the crying of the gulls are all around.

Gaby showed me his shell collection as I sat on the beach. The shells
were so light but so strong, tense with smooth concentric polished circles
or matted into a rough finish, curved on the inside with a silky splendour.
He placed them one by one on the palm of my hand. He loved them and
was proud of having gathered them. Joshua had made his own, less
systematic, collection, in which the category of the shell had been
interpreted more broadly. Scraps of interesting wood and pebbles were
mixed in with shells, half-shells and, the pride of the exhibition, a crab's
claw. The pincher could be moved in and out with satisfying results. I
returned the items in the collection one by one to Joshua, enclosing each
within my fist, which he had to open. He did this with grave concentra-
tion, until the claw came and nipped him.

As we criss-crossed the island in various directions, I wondered how
long it would take a blind person to get to know the island by the terrain
only. After a few walks, I recognized the place where the path turned
into the forest, crossing a rocky patch and then a wooden bridge. I
remembered how I had walked right around Holy Island, off the
Northumberland coast, accompanied by a sighted friend, but guided by
the steady prevailing wind. I could tell when we were half-way round,
three-quarters of the way round and so on, by the direction of the wind.
If I had had a tactile compass, I could even have told if the direction of
the wind had changed.

On one of the beaches on North Koster, the sea was completely
still. There was not even the slightest sound of lapping, and I located
the water with my cane rather than through hearing it. The family said
it was an inlet, almost enclosed, and a very quiet sea. I wondered
whether there would be a characteristic sound of each bay and inlet,
whether perhaps the sea would sound different on the eastern side of
the island. Would a blind person be able to recognize the general area
of the coast by the sound? The forest of conifers not only smelt
different; they sounded different as well. The wind in the pines

breathed and whistled but deciduous trees such as the oaks and the elms rustled and roared.

Losing the House   *12 August 1991*

The rest of the family had gone sailing around the Koster islands and were to be out all day. I worked indoors for a while, then went outside to see if the chairs and tables on the patio area were dry yet. There had been rain overnight and when I had tested the furniture earlier in the day, it was still dripping. Now it was nearly dry but the breeze was cool. Was the sun shining and if so, where? I worked my way around the edge of the patio, but it was all cool.

Yesterday, I had discovered that about twenty metres from the house there was another set of chairs around a table. It wasn't far from the annexe in which some of the children were sleeping. Marilyn had been sitting there reading and had called to me. Following her voice, I had discovered the garden bench where she sat. Maybe the sun would be shining there.

I went through the house and out of the side door, because this was the way I had gone to the place then. I set off without the cane, walking in what I guessed to be the same direction as yesterday and counting my steps.

After ten paces I stopped. The chairs could not be far away but it suddenly occurred to me that the property had no fence. Suppose I miscalculated slightly. The ground was rough with no distinctive markings. I went forward cautiously another five or six steps and stopped again. This must be the place. Why hadn't I brought my cane? I could have swished it round in a circle at least twelve feet in diameter. As it was, the table might be no more than a step away. Left or right? I took a few paces to the right. I had now walked in the shape of an L. Turning completely around, I retraced the few steps to the top of the L and continued, making it into a T. Still no chairs or table. But I could feel the sunshine. I would go back to the house, get the cane and try again.

At the head of the T I paused and listened. I must now be facing the house. The annexe must be on my left. The trees breathed heavily all around me, creating a rustly roof. I could not detect any particular pattern, as if there might be a gap where the house was. Why could I not sense the presence of so large an object? I clapped my hands but there did not seem to be an echo. I was obviously within shouting distance of the house but there was no one home. If I got lost, I could just sit down and wait. But it would be a long wait – it could not be more than eleven o'clock in the morning and the yacht would be out all day. 'Don't expect us back until after ten!' they had shouted cheerfully as they disappeared. I thought of the flask of hot coffee Marilyn had left for me, the beer in the fridge and my book waiting in the tape recorder. No, this was silly. The house was obviously right in front of me.

I stepped out briskly, counting the steps. The soles of my feet seemed to pick up every pebble, every fallen pine cone in the hope of remembering a pattern. Ten, fifteen, twenty steps and I stopped. I had gone further than before. Somehow I had missed it. Why had I been so careless as to walk the top of the T and back again? Why had I not made one outward journey, stopped and returned upon my tracks immediately to get the cane? I listened carefully. The distant sea was murmuring and there was the buzz of a small motor bike passing nearby. Should I call out?

I stooped down and picked up a handful of pebbles and fir-cones. I must remember which way I had come, otherwise I really would be lost. I threw the pebbles and fir-cones one by one in different directions. Some landed noiselessly. Some dropped on the ground with a soft thud, falling into grass or bracken. One or two struck something. The wooden house would sound hollow. A tree trunk would sound solid. Should I throw a bit harder? I didn't want to break a window. I must remember which way I had just come. The house must be on the right.

I moved to the right and encountered a fence. I had never met this fence before. Where on earth was I? Had I somehow got as far as a nearby property? Surely not. But this was not the annexe. I moved two or three feet along the fence and met a chair. On the chair was a cake of soap. Now I remembered.

Richard and Kate, who owned the house, had built an outside shower during the summer. It was served by a hosepipe running from the laundry. This must be it. Imogen and Marilyn had been using the shower every day, but the younger children and I had been washing in the laundry. House, annexe and shower must form three points of a circle.

From a post ran a clothes line. The sun was warm now on my face and the clothes were drying fast. Trailing my fingers along the line I followed it, expecting it to lead to the house. It finished at a tree. The tree went nowhere but up. This was no good; I had better go back to the shower.

It was now a matter of more or less random forays. I would go in and out away from the shower in various directions and see what happened. Off I went. Five, ten paces. There was a handrail, a banister, up a flight of steps. On the far side of the steps was the familiar wall of the house from which I had set out. I had always come down the steps on the house-wall side; I had never noticed that on the other side there was a banister. That made sense. The shower was just behind the back of the house. I was home. But where was the garden furniture?

I went into the house and got the white cane and set out again, walking in the original direction, counting the steps and swinging the cane as widely as I could from side to side so as to cover as much terrain as possible. It was amazing how the cane increased my power. Before, I was like an insect without antennae, a cat without whiskers. Now I felt armed. I could do in one sweep what it would have taken me lots of confusing criss-crossings to do before. I could do it without getting lost, because the cane revealed contours which the isolated feet could not. Crack! There it was; the mysterious table and beside it the bench and the chairs. The wooden slats were warm with the morning sun. As I sat down, I noticed that the palms of my hands were moist. I did not want to go through all that again. I carefully arranged the bench so that it pointed towards the house, and made the journey from house to bench several times feeling, in a funny sort of way, both more confident and more isolated each time.

Suddenly, I did not want to be sitting out there on the bench in the sunshine. I wanted to have the familiar feel of the patio under my feet and the front door handle only an arm's length away. Sooner or later during the day, the sun would get round there. I could wait. The coffee was hot and the beer was cold. I returned to the patio and started reading.

The day passed happily. In the evening, everyone returned, full of exciting stories about their sailing adventures. I made no reference to my own adventure.

Later in the week, Richard came from Oslo to visit us. He and Marilyn, with a few children, sat on the patio chatting.

'So they left you behind, did they?' asked Richard. 'What did you do all day?' I explained that I had mainly sat on the patio reading and sleeping.

Marilyn said, 'But the sun doesn't come round here until the middle of the afternoon. Why didn't you use the other set of chairs over there?'

'Oh,' I said, 'I did find them, but I was afraid of getting lost, or losing the house, not being able to get back to the house.' I could sense that they were both staring at me with surprise.

'Yes,' said Marilyn gently, 'but it's only a few feet away'.

'It would be OK,' I explained, 'if the house had a fence around it. Without a fence, I somehow felt that if I were to miss it or forget which way the house was I might wander off into the forest or get disorientated.' There was a pause. Richard and Marilyn were considering this.

'I see what you mean,' she said softly, 'but it's so hard to really take it in.'

Thunder over Koster   *13 August 1991*

The slow Scandinavian sun had gone down in a glory of colour. It must have been remarkable, because even Thomas said 'Cor!' They described it to me. The clouds were piled up on banks, as if they were upside down, in layers ranging from red and gold through the purest light green and grey-blue. It was very still. The sun sets silently; the planet turns smoothly.

Now at last they were all in bed. I had told the final story and Marilyn had done the final late-night round with the mosquito repellent. Imogen and I were going through one of her philosophy texts when she exclaimed 'What was that? Something's happened! There it is again – wow! What a flash!' She turned to the window.

'It's lightning,' Marilyn said. 'It must be. It must be sheet lightning. But there's no sound, no thunder. Now there's a whole series of them – the whole island is lit up. I can't see any forks or sheets of lightning; just the flash itself.'

'I'm going to listen,' I said, moving to the door and stepping outside. The night was completely still. There was no breeze, no gulls; even the sea had shrunk to a quiet murmur. I made myself comfortable leaning on the wall and waited. Occasionally, Imogen and Marilyn called out 'It's still flashing, even brighter.' I waited. I wanted to hear the first sound.

There was something, but what? Was it a sound or just a tremor in the air? Had I heard it or felt it? Did it come from above or below? It was a tremor, but whether on the earth or the air I could not say.

It came again, very deep and echoey, a distant door opening on silent hinges, revealing for a moment a huge vaulted chamber, and then closing just as silently. It was as though the lid had been lifted momentarily from a profound cavern within which could be heard the deep shaking of the surge. The lid was replaced without a sound, without an effort, and the island waited breathlessly.

Far away, perhaps on the mainland, perhaps up in the mountains, there were muffled drums. I thought of the passage in *The Lord of the Rings* where deep inside the mountains Gandalf and his party heard the muffled drums of the approaching Orcs. It was so distant that it was sure to pass us by. Perhaps that was why there had been flashes without any visible stroke of lightning: it was too distant. They were looking for us but they would not find us. They were too far away.

But now the tremor had grown to a murmur and the murmur into a grumble. It had a bouncy quality, as if huge muffled stones were being rolled down vast fields. I thought of Thor and of the ancient people, listening long ago and waiting.

Suddenly the thunder sprang. The muffled stones had been a manoeuvre to distract my attention while the main force of the enemy stole up unnoticed. A long peal of thunder disturbed the air, no longer low upon the distant fields but at a height, as if rising up to attack. The trees stirred uneasily. Waves of wind broke across the tree-tops, coming closer then fizzing over the house, leaving a swirling trail of restlessness behind. The wind carried a fragrance in it, the scent of the heather, of seaweed and salt, the aroma of the fir trees. The first drops of rain fell on my face and pattered on the wooden patio. I could hear the storm coming across the island. There was a rush of wind and I thought of Dorothy's house in Kansas being carried up by the tornado. Suddenly the thunder and the rain seemed to squash the house flat and hurl it, pinned to the surface of the island.

Everything was alive. Someone was hitting the sky with a huge mallet. The sky was made of canvas or hide. It flapped and cracked as it was hit again and again. Then the sky was no longer canvas but metal. Thor's hammer flew across its corrugated surface, breaking it open with a triumphant crash and the rain came down in a torrent.

I stepped hastily back indoors. 'That was a beauty!' cried Imogen.

'Are you ready for more coffee?' asked Marilyn.

'No,' I said, 'I'm going out the back to listen.'

On the side or back of the house was a covered porch, open on one side. The roof of this little porch was hammered by the rain while high above (but not too high) the roof of the world was hammered by Thor. There were two levels; one was consistent and steady like the drone of the bagpipes while the other was broken into phrases, like the melody line of a vast symphony for cello and percussion.

As suddenly as it had started, it faded. The mighty conductor lowered the baton. The triple f on the score turned to the double and a single. The belt of thunder had passed over the island and was moving away. As if it could not bear to be left behind, the rain followed.

As the clattering on the roof died way, a curtain was lifted upon the surrounding woodland. All other sound but that of the thunder itself had been blanketed out by the rain on the roof, but now the rest of the world became audible. It fell on the nearby annexe roof with a sharp patter; the trees were waving sodden arms and hissing with pleasure. The ground for yards around was sucking and tinkling as thousands of blades of grass gulped in the drops. Now the roofs were silent and the gurgling began. Down the drainpipes the disappearing water gushed in a mad cascade of escape. Now the gurgling finished and the dripping began. They were everywhere – big drops, little drops, slow drops, fast drops, dripping interrupted by small splashes as if other drops couldn't wait to drip. The trees were dripping like dogs shaking themselves in the final puffs of wind.

Then it was all gone. The muffled drums of departure in the sky must now be heard as a distant warning by some other island further along the coast. A final undefeated drop made an occasional ping on a metal seat somewhere.

I went back inside. The coffee was still hot.

Crabs   *17 August 1991*

By the jetty on Koster was a little shop selling fish and seafood. Marilyn left the children buying ice-cream at the general store and walked along the front towards the shop. It was closed and as we hovered outside the front door, hoping for some indication of an opening hour, a man greeted us. Marilyn had spent six months learning Norwegian, only to discover that the language spoken on the island was Swedish. Nevertheless, the languages are very similar, and she was doing remarkably well. There was a brief exchange, then Marilyn said 'He wants us to jump on his bike. I think he is going to take us to where we can get some crabs.' Leading me forward, she placed my hand on the edge of a large wooden tray.

'What? On here?' I cried, not certain what she meant. 'Me as well?'

'Yes, of course, come on! I'm on already.' The motor bike was already revved up as I leapt on to the tray, hanging my legs over the side and holding on for dear life. I was so busy trying not to be thrown off that I could not really work out if I was being carried on the front or the back of the machine.

We roared along and then there were cries of surprise from the children, who greeted us with astonishment.

'Stop! Where are you going? Come back!' they cried, as we swept past them.

'We don't know . . . we're off to get some crabs . . . see you later!' Marilyn and I shouted between screams of laughter.

The children's shouting receded into the distance as we tore up a hillside, bumping over the dirt track, around a corner and down a long slope. We seemed to be coming into a part of the island we had not visited before. Was he taking us to another shop, or was he perhaps a fisherman?

Abruptly, the motorbike stopped and we jumped off. We were led through some sort of shed rich with all sorts of fishy goods and out on to a jetty, beneath which could be heard the lapping of the waves. Marilyn exclaimed 'Good gracious! They're still alive,' and now we were back inside the shed being offered mackerel as well as crab. Marilyn bartered briskly in a mixture of Norwegian, English, Swedish and fingers, and out we came into the sunlight to be greeted by the children, delighted and relieved to have found us. They had run all the way, half laughing, half crying. Their mood of relieved indignation soon turned to joy when the fisherman offered them a ride back. All three of them jumped aboard with whoops of glee and off they went. Now it was our turn to wave and shout goodbyes. The clamour travelled up the hill and disappeared as Marilyn and I, arm in arm, walked happily home through the trees, swinging a rather alarmingly full bag of fish and crabs.

I gathered that the crabs had been kept alive in a basket hanging from the jetty by a rope. The fisherman had simply pulled it up and popped four of his liveliest specimens into a bag. The amount of bashing, smashing and cursing did not seem proportionate to the minute quantities of crab meat which adorned the supper salad, and the younger members of the family ate with a certain air of reserve. The smooth crab paste in jars from the supermarket seemed worlds away, but if they did not eat up, there was a threat of more smashing and bashing tomorrow. Anyway, the bike ride had been an adventure for everyone.

Princess of Scandinavia   *19 August 1991*

We were homeward bound. There was the familiar clanking as the car rolled down the ramp into the vessel. The *Princess* was the sister of the *Prince* and the layout was almost identical. The children noisily banged on the doors of the cabins with the same numbers we had had before and were dragged off by embarrassed parents.

One thing was different: the sea was up. The outward voyage had been as smooth as a table; this time the ship developed quite a roll. It was interesting walking uphill and downdale but a little unpredictable. Tom was quite unaffected, but the rest of the family soon felt slightly strange.

The cabins were neatly equipped with plastic bags and soon the children rushed off to the cinema, each with a bag in a pocket. They quickly returned, crying with fascinated horror that someone had been sick in the corridor. 'Don't be so silly!' said Marilyn, always resourceful. 'Just go round the other way.'

The cabin did not include a toilet, so I asked Thomas to help me learn the route to the nearest public washroom. Leaving the cabin, we turned right, walking down a corridor past cabin doors. A handrail made it easy to keep steady. The corridor turned left at an angle of forty-five degrees. The first opening on the right was a bulkhead through which we had to step. We were now in another long corridor which finished with a second bulkhead and we stepped into some kind of open space. Thomas taught me to locate the first pillar, then the second, and so we came to the door to the gents' washroom in the far left-hand corner.

Could I learn it so that even if I came out in the middle of the night alone I could find my way there and back?

Thomas stayed behind, watching but offering no help, as I retraced our steps. I walked rapidly so as to keep the pattern in my mind. In my right hand was the cane; with my left hand I trailed a finger along the handrail where there was one. In my mind was a map of the area and I was a small red light moving along it. I watched the red light. It paused at the first column and again at the second. It missed the bulkhead the first time by going too far to the right, but quickly found it by tracking left along the wall through the bulkhead. Down the long corridor, past many doors. The second bulkhead and a T junction. Left or right? Left, of course, provided there was soon a forty-five degree angle to the right. There was. I must be nearly there. I must not overshoot my cabin. There were many doors. Must be nearly there. Start feeling the cabin door handles. Gently. Don't rattle them in case someone thinks you are trying to get in. Sleepy passenger in night-dress finds confused blind man trying to get in at three in the morning. Where was the door handle around which I had tied the handkerchief? Had someone stolen the handkerchief? Then I would be sunk. No, here it is. I untied the handkerchief, put it in my pocket and went in. Two more practice runs, the first with Thomas, the second without him. Now I was confident I could do it.

I decided to have an early night, and lay on the comfortable bunk enjoying the swaying of the cabin, but feeling rather glad that I wasn't walking up and down the deck. Now there were two ways I could tell the ship was pitching and tossing slightly. First, I could feel the drag of my body on the bed; it was just enough to make me wonder if I was going to slip an inch or two. Then it would turn and I would feel the drag in the other direction. Secondly, everything in the cabin was a little noisier than on the outward voyage. There was more creaking and shuddering, and now and then the cabin seemed to hesitate, as if not quite sure which way to go. All the time the deep living purr of the ship itself seemed to say 'Seas come and go, but I am always here. I shall continue my appointed way.'

In the morning, I went with Thomas, Lizzie and Gaby for an early breakfast. The restaurant offered a most interesting experience. It rattled. Every cup on the table rattled on its saucer and every spoon in its bowl. The loose cutlery kept chattering as if to say 'Here we are!' The edge of the table, usually marked only by where voices came from, was not where the clattering stopped. Beyond our table, other tables were picked out, not by the murmur of conversation but by becoming little tinkling islands. The light fixtures on the ceiling and on the walls vibrated gently and the furthest trolley was jangling all over. At the far end of the cafeteria the long service hatch was pulsating, and (I think it was the coffee dispenser) there was a lovely tattoo where a couple of sheets of metal were in conversation.

It was as if the whole room was talking. Everything was saying 'We don't have to wait for rain – we can do this by ourselves.'

Afterwards, I remarked to a member of the family 'Wasn't it nice the way it rattled in the restaurant?'

'Rattled?' came the reply. 'What do you mean rattled? I didn't notice any rattling.' Sighted people are strange. I sometimes wonder just what sort of a world they live in.

Arriving home after a four-hour car drive from Harwich, Lizzie rushed up the stairs shouting 'I'm going to say hello to my room.' I hurried after her. She ran across the landing and threw open the door of her room. 'Hello room!' she cried in delight.

I understood that. Perhaps sighted people are not so strange after all.

'Thou Shalt Touch'   *23 August 1991*

Marilyn and I had been invited to attend the fifth exhibition of sculpture from blind and sighted artists in Kortenhoef, near Amsterdam, sponsored by the College Trust. The exhibition was located in and around the village church, including the vestry, the surrounding lawns and approaches, the apple orchard and the tent pitched next door. Exhibits ranged in size from those smaller than the human hand to some so huge I could hardly reach the top. They were made of peat and light bulbs, of bronze and clay, wood and marble, rubber, papier-mâché and plastic.

I explored them, a dozen or so at a time. In the intervals I sat in the garden under a vine drinking coffee or beer, talking with my hosts, with the artists or with visitors to the exhibition. Several of the artists were from the eastern part of Germany and two or three were from Russia, but most were from the Netherlands.

We agreed that there is a difference between the way blind and sighted people approach both life and art. Sighted people begin with the whole and then go on to the details. They are first general and then particular. Blind people go the opposite way. They begin with detail and then advance to the whole. Each must make a certain effort in order to empathize with the other. It is difficult for sighted people ever to begin with the details, for the general overview which sight provides has already robbed the hands of their distinctive approach through the particular.

What would it be, to know life through its particularities? The world of blind people is so tiny, so particular, that sighted people can hardly imagine it. On the other hand, to begin with detail is curious, because you do not know if it is a detail until you go beyond it. It is, at first, a whole in that it is all the finger can encompass, or the hand can touch at once. It only becomes a detail as a result of further exploration, and even after a good deal of exploration it may still not be clear what it is a detail of.

Because the sighted person examining a sculpture takes it in all at once, there is a tendency towards premature generalization. The sighted person, having looked at the statue for a few moments, often wants to know what it is or what it is called. The entire thing has to be summed up in some way. For the blind person, on the other hand, detail leads to detail and the pleasure of the hand is autonomous. There is a pleasure in discovering that the two hands experience similar undulating surfaces if placed at just this angle, and there is a pleasure in running the fingers round and round this particular edge, past the place where it widens out, ending again and again at that fascinating point.

In the case of those sculptures which were most obviously designed to be touched, they gave themselves to the hand and the hand did not need the head in order to understand them. Sometimes, having explored an item, it was interesting to read the braille title. It was, of course, in Dutch and since I do not know Dutch the meaning was usually unclear, but I could at least say the title. It was like giving the statue a name. This was a form of affirmation, even though I did not know what the name meant. Nevertheless, it is true that the hand can sometimes fail to grasp the intention of the whole structure, although I am inclined to think that in such cases the item was not really made with touch as the first priority.

226

There was one particularly cunning piece of work. It was in the form of an upright cigar, or rounded canoe, with several oval-shaped holes through which various other structures were discovered. These consisted of the same basic shape but made in different materials and presented in different sizes and positions. In the deeper recesses they could only be reached by hand. It was a bit like feeling into someone's body.

Many of the exhibits seemed to be bodies or parts of bodies. This was true not only of those statues which were obviously lovers intertwined, but of many of the more abstract shapes. An upright wooden statue standing about twenty centimetres tall reminded me of a human foot. Next to it, a piece of marble, so wonderfully curved, was like a Venus de Milo which had lost legs and breasts as well as arms, and yet was inexpressibly feminine. Perhaps it's just me, but there was something rather exhausting about the continual bodily inspection which close tactile examination of these statues seemed to require.

Beyond Touch   *24 August 1991*

The pastor in charge of the exhibition took me to the marble altar in his church. 'I imagine,' he said, 'that this is a bit like the altar in Iona Abbey which you described in your book *Touching the Rock*.' It was very beautiful indeed; but it did not have those scratch marks or scarred indentations which broke the smooth surface of the Iona altar and gave one that strange feeling of encountering the ultimate beneath the beautiful.

I mentioned this to Henk, who told me he had been discussing with several sculptors the problems of representing the ineffable to touch, of enabling touch to realize that it cannot grasp the transcendent. He had thought about creating a large circular serving dish from bronze. It would be textured or patterned, except for the centre which would be smooth but just out of reach. You would be able to reach to where the patterning stopped and the surface became smooth but you would not be able to reach into the very centre. As he pointed out, there were problems in this. It could not be adapted for the different lengths of the arm, and without sight it is difficult to tell how you would know, as you went around the large plate exploring it, that there was an unreachable centre part.

Nevertheless, the idea is intriguing. It is not difficult to create a sense of the mysterious visually. Every cathedral does it, with long lines of pillars disappearing into mysterious shadows intersected by shafts of coloured light. Moreover, there are some things which simply cannot be looked at, like the sun, or things cloaked in darkness. This gives rise to the idea that it is impossible to gaze upon God, or that God is cloaked in deep darkness, one who is hidden. There are indeed some visual art forms which are particularly appropriate to convey the transcendent. One thinks of stained glass, and of the synagogue windows by Marc Chagal, to say nothing of the wonderful rose window in Chartres. What corresponds to this in the world of touch?

At first grasp, we might suppose that touch was essentially intimate and explicit, rather than distant and ineffable. How can that which has been brought within your grasp convey the elusive? Perhaps one could make use of temperature? The hand draws back from heat just as the eye from excessive brightness. What about a large bronze plate which got hotter as you explored towards its centre? What about using slight electric shocks to indicate the limit of acceptable touch? Perhaps one could feel in towards a hole, which simply fell away from the hand. Perhaps one could make use of the reach of the arm, which has an obvious limit. What about a vessel, the bottom of which cannot be reached?

Such ideas may present some possibilities but I have my doubts. When your hand meets something hot, or receives a slight electric shock, you draw away and say 'ouch'. When you stand under the full radiance of the sun there is a sense of majesty, of power greater than the capacity of the human eye to comprehend. The tactile experiences just described are surely rather trivial in comparison. They do not convey the sense of the serenity of the one who dwells in unapproachable light, whom no one has seen nor can see. The visual metaphors seem to have the advantage. As for putting one's arm into a barrel or an urn, the bottom of which cannot be reached, this is just annoying, especially if you have dropped something in it. The hand is frustrated rather than transcended. The difference in religious terms is all important.

We are trying to be too clever. Someone sent me a wooden ring about five centimetres in diameter. It came wrapped in a piece of paper upon which were written the words 'Hold infinity in the palm of your hand'. Hold this pebble. This shell: hold it to your ear and be silent. Let the grains of sand run between your fingers, on and on. Pick up another handful and squeeze it tight until the grains escape between your fingers and your hand is empty. Do it again and again. Leave your house and step outside. You can see nothing, but it does not matter. Within there are limits; outside, there are no limits. You sense the boundless space, the movements of air coming from a free and inexhaustible place, and then you go back inside, into the warmth and intimacy of human habitation, with the lingering odours of cooking and sleeping. Your body knows the finite and the infinite. God does not dwell only in houses made with hands. Hold to your heart the body of this child. Yes, the sense of touch can reveal the mysterious, that which is beyond.

To some extent, art can replicate these experiences. I run my hands around this crystal ball, this solid sphere of glass. There is absolutely no detail. There is, in a sense, nothing to hold on to yet I feel as if I could hold it for ever. I would like to examine a one-track labyrinth made in wood, small enough for the hand. That might suggest similar impressions.

One of the items in the exhibition was a single stone of polished marble, shaped like a kidney or a bean. It was about thirty centimetres long. I imagined it being found on the surface of the moon. It would be like the megalith discovered by the astronauts in *Space Odyssey – 2001*: obviously a work of intelligence when seen against the lunar surface. Although intended by a shaping mind, the stone remains enigmatic; it is squat, compact, self-contained and determined to give little or nothing away. It is as old as eternity and will remain when these hands of mine which rest upon its fascinating surface have long turned to dust.

Touch Me   *25 August 1991*

One of the participants in the exhibition was introduced to me.

'Are you a sculptor?' I asked.

'Not exactly,' he replied. 'I make acoustic architecture, sonic structures.'

'You mean music?'

'Not exactly, although music may have these qualities. I make acoustic patterns which pick up a certain space, which enable the listener to grasp the space. It is a way of extending perception for the blind, but it also has much to offer the sighted. Perhaps you will listen to my modest attempt later in the day.'

Henk explained that between three and four o'clock every afternoon a group of sound sculptors would use the church bell to create a noise.

At three o'clock the noise began. From the church tower there came a high-pitched continuous sound, less strident than a siren, but more metallic than a flute. It sounded a little like the noise a saw makes when played with a violin bow, except it maintained a level pitch and seemed to be composed of thousands of pitter patters, like vibrations. The sound rose and fell a little, like a train whistle, with the wind, and depending on where one stood. It was not particularly loud, but one could not fail to notice it. Henk told me that depending on the direction of the wind it could be heard for five kilometres.

'Would you like to climb up into the tower and meet the performers?'

We climbed together. At first the circular stone stairway was broad and easy. After several flights and a small landing we entered upon a smaller stone staircase, winding more steeply. Stone then seemed to give way to wood, and I was ducking beneath beams to find the first step of a short staircase which led to an area with a rough wooden floor. Now the sound of the ringing was very close. I began to mount a wooden ladder. It had twenty or twenty-five rungs and brought me out right beneath the huge early-fifteenth-century bell. Two or three men were sitting in the belfry around the bell, striking the outside of it with heavy mallets. A mallet was thrust into my hand.

'Don't your wrists get tired after an hour of this?'

'Yes, but we have two shifts and we keep changing. If you climb up a little higher you can feel the bell itself.'

I was now head and shoulders within the bell. It was about two metres in diameter. I could not reach the far side without losing my balance, but I could grasp the tongue of the bell which was hanging beside me. The lump on the end was as large as a human head. I rested my hands on the bell. It was vibrating violently. I wondered foolishly if I could muffle it a little by the pressure of my hand but hard as I pressed it made no difference. The sound architects explained that they had a device for measuring the level of sound. If it dropped too low, they knew they were getting tired and would increase their efforts.

Since I was actually inside the bell, the sound had no particular point of origin. It came from everywhere. It was hard to tell if it was inside my head or outside. Only my hands on the bell and my feet on the rung of the ladder held me to the world. I felt as if my brain was floating away. I made my way down, slowly and carefully, noticing how the world returned as the sound of the bell grew more faint.

In the churchyard, Henk approached me. Taking my fingers he placed them in a pile of powder which he held in his hand.

'What do you think this is?' he asked.

I felt it carefully between finger and thumb. It was the softest of powdery substances, a bit like talcum powder. It could have been a very fine white flour. There was a slightly moist quality; it clung to the skin, but perhaps that was only because it was so fine.

'Flour?' I asked.

'Far from it!' he laughed, taking me a few steps to where one of the sculptors was at work. I had to stoop slightly as he laid my hand in a

230

trench a couple of inches wide, full of this powder. 'It is powder from the marble; it is marble dust.'

Lying on the ground was a large block of the finest quality marble. It was perhaps just over a metre long, a block some sixty to seventy centimetres deep. A trough was being cut across it so as to divide it into two sections. An electric drill had been used, and the powder was the result. The sculptor pointed out the three stages of the process. First, there was the rough cutting of the block, and then the flat but slightly rough surfaces where it had been smoothed off. Finally there was the powder. It was remarkable to think that something so hard and firm could be reduced to this texture.

Postscript: The Meaning of Blindness

In this book, an attempt has been made to interpret blindness through a series of diary entries. No other form could have expressed the immediacy and the fragmentary character of this experience. The sporadic nature of the entries indicates both the repetition of a pain which never seems to heal and the discovery of a healing which is so slow as to be almost unnoticed.

The book's main themes are the finding of something solid and permanent on the far side of despair and a change in the character of consciousness. There is something urgent and intense about trying to touch a rock when you are being swept away, but from that safer place it is possible to survey the experience from a wider perspective. What emerges is a sort of philosophy, theology and sociology of blindness. It is, of course, in fragments, and perhaps it always will be.

I have constructed two points of view towards consciousness. There is a crack in consciousness and there is a fall into consciousness. In the first case, consciousness represents that which is blindingly obvious. Day-by-day reality in the only society I know, that of late industrial modernity, is so obvious that it becomes invisible. You only notice the windscreen when a crack develops in it, and the taken-for-granted nature of everyday life late in the twentieth century is only challenged by some profound disaster. This may be of a personal or a social nature. In fact, the surface of this consciousness, both socially and subjectively, is worn thin in many places, and can fracture quite easily. Sometimes, a little education can do it. The purpose of loss, the character of revelation and the role of education is to push people down these cracks. Once you are half-way down a crack you realize that the consciousness which now, for the first time, you begin to see from beneath, is actually a false consciousness. You then realize that you have looked and looked but never seen, seen but never perceived,

232

perceived but never understood, understood but never repented, repented but never acted.

You slip through the crack. You fall. You scream. Somehow or other, you land, only to find that you have fallen into consciousness. Why is it that the path from one consciousness to another is by way of this inversion? There is no direct path. There is a long detour, a stripping off, a laying bare, a circuitous track by means of which we discover that in losing everything, not everything is lost, that in abandonment, not everything is abandoned, that in losing we find and in dying we live.

Here we come to a curious feature of this inversion, this recoil of consciousness upon itself. Whereas the intention of the surface consciousness is individualizing, its reality is social. The intention of the deeper consciousness is social and economic but it is experienced as a spirituality which integrates one with all. The subjectivity of the surface consciousness is aware of its own thoughts and emotions, its own ambitions and possessions; it does not realize that it is but a mirror. When the mirror cracks and you go through it, you look back on a different world.

My interpretation of blindness has led me from archetypes to socio-economic phenomenology. The first phase of the interpretation was regression into the archetype; the second phase of the interpretation was a return with the archetype into the present and future of our society. In other words, the symbols with which I have tried to interpret blindness must not be interpreted archaically, romantically or nostalgically, but dynamically, futuristically and historically. In speaking of that which lies beyond light and darkness, or of the terrible gift, or of finding fulfilment in praise, I have not wished to clothe the nakedness of the blind condition in the comforting mythologies of a former age.

We are facing in our time an immense despiritualization of life, a process in which human beings and things are all being turned into commodities. By way of reaction there is a yearning for spiritual renewal, which expresses itself in all kinds of excitable inwardness, cognitive hardness and cosmic mysticism. In order to make creative use of the experience of blindness, however, it is necessary to confront directly the socio-economic character of this despiritualization. In its intimacy, its openness, its weakness and its vulnerability, blindness can offer a sort of archetype of the future. Blindness offers this in many ways, not only in itself but also through awakening the tactile and acoustic worlds. It can be a way, and I myself have only partially realized this, of understanding and overcoming the great historic divisions of humanity into the weak and the strong, those in wealth and those in poverty, those in sickness and those in health. To grasp this is to turn the stigma of blindness into a calling, from stigma to stigmata. The same is true of any experience of human weakness, which is why the Kingdom of God is to be found amongst children and amongst the poor.

Some symbols are like the ashes of a dying fire. They warm your private heart in your declining years. Others are like fuel – they drive the fire forward so that it leaps higher and higher and consumes everything. Perhaps sight can also be a fuel. Perhaps anything can. I do not know. I can only report on one person's journey. For me, to be grasped by blindness is to be grasped by a demand for a more mutual humanity, and in that grasp to feel the tug of the future.

By the same author

In the Beginning there was Darkness, SCM Press, 2001
Utopian Whispers: Moral, Religious and Spiritual Values in Schools,
   Religious and Moral Education Press, 1998
Mishmash: Religious Education in a Multicultural Britain, A Study
   in Metaphor, University of Birmingham and the Christian Education
   Movement, 1991
Hellenistic Magic and the Synoptic Tradition, SCM Press, 1975
Sense and Nonsense about God, SCM Press, 1974